ANATOMISTS AND EPONYMS

The Spirit of Anatomy Past

KO Gilliland
RL Montgomery

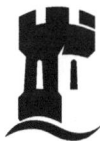

Nottingham
University Press

First published by Nottingham University Press
This reissued original edition published 2023 by 5m Books Ltd www.5mbooks.com

British Library Cataloguing in Publication Data
Anatomists and Eponyms: The Spirit of Anatomy Past

ISBN 9781789182712

Disclaimer

Every reasonable effort has been made to ensure that the material in this book is true, correct, complete
and appropriate at the time of writing. Nevertheless the publishers and the author do not accept
responsibility for any omission or error, or for any injury, damage, loss or financial consequences
arising from the use of the book. Views expressed in the articles are those of the author and not of the
Editor or Publisher.

With special thanks to Meredith Browne for permission to use images from "The Alphabet of Anatomical
Eponyms" ©Meredith Browne http://meredithbrowne.weebly.com/alphabet-of-anatomical-eponyms.html

Cover image: ©Meredith Browne

Typeset by Nottingham University Press, Nottingham

EU GPSR Authorised Representative
LOGOS EUROPE, 9 rue Nicolas Poussin, 17000, LA ROCHELLE, France
E-mail: Contact@logoseurope.eu

CONTENTS

FOREWORD

Most of us learned about the Achilles tendon and the cell's Golgi apparatus in high school biology, but what was so significant about Achilles and who was Camillo Golgi? Maybe you are surprised that the Eustachian tube is named after a scientist named Bartolomeo Eustachi and that the Fallopian tube was identified by a man named Gabriele Falloppio? Many parts of the human body – from visible protuberances on bones to microscopic cells within glands – bear the names of famous anatomists, physicians, and even mythological characters. Whether it was Galen of ancient Rome, Vesalius of medieval Italy, or John Hunter of late 18th-century England, we owe much of our current understanding of the human body to scientists of the past.

An **eponym** is a person whose name is, or is thought to be, the source of the name of something, such as a city, country, era, or in this case anatomical structure. The older traditional human anatomical textbooks included numerous anatomical eponyms. This practice was a desire to perpetuate the memory of original investigators by associating their names with the anatomical structures that they discovered. The current trends in most medical school curricula have reduced the subject matter in human anatomy to its barest essentials with the elimination of most eponyms. Instead, structures are identified only by descriptive scientific terms. Both students and teachers are now therefore deprived of learning the history associated with many of the former great anatomists.

The objective of this book is to introduce eponyms for which common anatomical structures are named. The eponyms included are related to some form of *normal* anatomy – gross anatomy, histology (microscopic anatomy or cell biology), neuroanatomy, and embryology (developmental anatomy). There was no intent to include eponyms associated with other basic science disciplines such as biochemistry, genetics, physiology, microbiology, immunology, or pharmacology. Nor was there any attempt to include eponyms associated with the numerous techniques, procedures, equipment, and nomenclature related to clinical sciences such as surgery, obstetrics and gynecology, pediatrics, psychiatry, radiology, the many subspecialties of medicine, or the numerous diseases of pathology. Only the more common eponyms associated with the various anatomical systems of the human body are included, with a focus on the normal rather than the abnormal state. The eponyms included are the ones which are still commonly used, which are often the subject of the quizzing of medical students in the clinics and operating rooms, and for which there often is no other descriptive term.

The authors wish to acknowledge Lippincott Williams & Wilkins/Wolters Kluwer Health for permission to use several images from *Anatomy as a Basis for Clinical Medicine*, 3rd edition, by E.C.B. Hall-Craggs (Williams, and Wilkins, 1995). The images used are of the dural venous sinuses (page 8), skin (28), breast (30), leg (33), atlas (34), hip (34), sternum (35 and 42), inguinal ligament (37 and 43), abdominal wall (39), thigh (40), forearm (41), brachial plexus (50), orbit (53), brainstem (65), rectum (85), duodenum (86), sagittal uterus (104), frontal pelvis (105), transverse pelvis (107), cochlear duct (111 and 113), nasal cavity (117), eyelid (118), and eye (119). All other images are property of the authors or are in the public domain.

HISTORY

EARLY ANATOMY

The cave paintings of the early Stone Age, approximately 30,000 years ago, depicted a simple knowledge of the anatomy of animals. The early civilisations of the Babylonians, Egyptians, Assyrians, Chinese, and Hindus contributed very little to our knowledge of human anatomy. Each of these cultures placed enormous religious restrictions against the dissection of the human body. Severe penalties were given to those individuals who disfigured or violated the "sanctity of the deceased human body."

The progress of medicine was stagnated not only by religious factors but also by man's fear and superstition of the dead. Ghosts associated with the dead were judged to be vengeful and vindictive. In order for medicine to advance, it was necessary for the profession to dissect and study the human body without the fear of ghosts and punishment from the church.

ANATOMY IN ANCIENT GREECE

500-200 B.C.

Alcmaeon (500 B.C.). Alcmaeon was probably the first individual to dissect a human body. He has been given credit for suggesting that the brain is the center of intelligence.

Hippocrates (460-377 B.C.). Hippocrates, the famous Greek physician, is often regarded as the father of medicine. The Hippocratic Oath taken by graduating medical students is a promise and duty to serve mankind. Hippocrates promoted the concept of four humors of the body which were associated with the blood (liver), yellow bile (gallbladder), phlegm (lungs), and melancholy or black bile (spleen). A balance of the four humors was associated with good health. This concept of four humors, even though totally incorrect, dominated medical theory for approximately 2,000 years. Hippocrates' knowledge of the human body was severely limited by the lack of dissections. The greatest contribution of Hippocrates was that he attributed diseases to natural causes rather than to the displeasures of the gods.

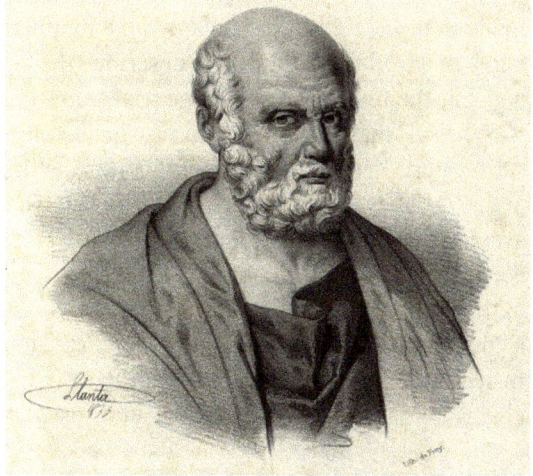

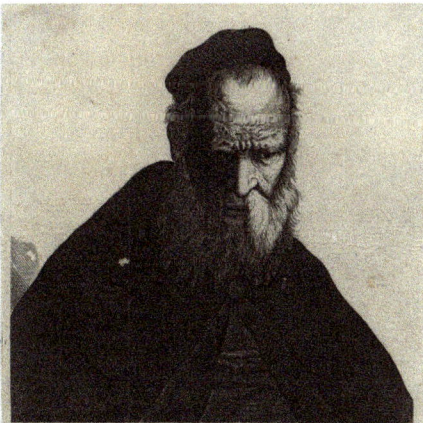

Al gran Rè uinciter vinto dall' ira
Questo gran saggia i documenti diede,
Mori, mà nel morir di fama herede,
Che non morirà mai lascò stagirea.

Aristotle (384-322 B.C.). Prior to Aristotle, anatomy was without substance. He is considered by many to be the first comparative anatomist of that particular era. Aristotle wrote the first known account of embryology and was the first to describe the development of the heart in the chick embryo. He has been credited with the naming of the aorta, contrasting the arteries and veins, and differentiating nerves from tendons. Although often called the father of comparative anatomy, Aristotle was also responsible for several erroneous anatomical concepts. He believed the heart to be the site of intelligence and the brain to be responsible for cooling the blood.

Herophilus (335-280 B.C.). Herophilus was the first individual to open the human body after death for the sole purpose of determining the cause of death and was a pioneer in dissecting human bodies in public. Fallopius even called him the "evangelist of the anatomists." The most significant discovery by Herophilus was made in the brain where he named the confluence of sinuses, which carries the name of torcular herophili. He described the brain as the location of intelligence and was the first to acknowledge nerves as either sensory or motor. Herophilus was the first man to name the furrow in the fourth ventricle, calling it the calamus scriptorius. In addition, Herophilus was the first to distinguish between arteries and veins and was probably the first to teach a female medical student. Serious accusations charged Herophilus with dissecting living humans. The first to accuse him was Celsus (42 B.C.-A.D. 37). Much later, an outstanding member of the early Christian Church, Tertullian (155-222), accused Herophilus of being a "butcher" who dissected 600 men in order to find out nature. The accusations made by both Celsus and Tertullian have never been proven and therefore will always remain nothing more than a curiosity.

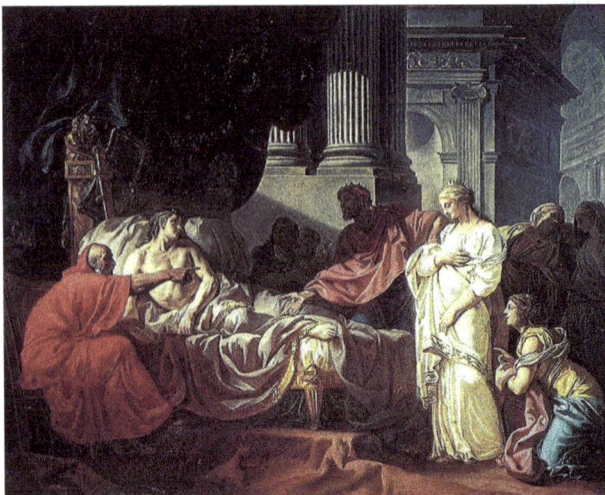

Erasistratus (310-250 B.C.). Erasistratus, who was presumed to be the grandson of Aristotle, dissected the human body publicly at the Alexandrian school. He was the first to catalogue both sensory and motor nerves and believed that the cerebrum was the site for intellect and all nervous functions. Erasistratus also studied the circulation in the human body; believed that pneuma, or vital air, was carried in the arteries; and placed the soul in the meninges. Several sources have indicated that both Herophilus and Erasistratus dissected the dead as well as the living (vivisection).

Claudius Galen
130-200

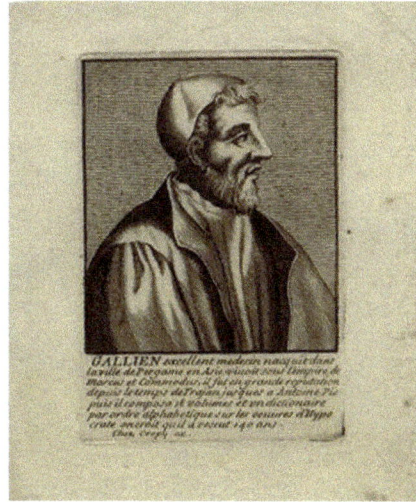

Galen was considered by many to be one of the greatest ancient physicians. His medical writings ruled the medical world for approximately 1500 years. His extended influence on the medical world was related to his prolific writings which were followed by a period in which human anatomical dissections were not permitted. To question Galen's writings became a heresy as he had become accepted as an infallible master. Galen made very few personal contributions to our knowledge of human anatomy. In fact, most of the human anatomy known by Galen was restricted to the skeleton and what he had observed in superficial wounds of the gladiators. Furthermore, his knowledge of the viscera was gained primarily from pigs, sheep, cats, dogs, horses, fish, monkeys and apes – not humans.

Galen probably dissected fewer than two human bodies as he was never given the permission to dissect the human body. Thus he perpetuated the four humors of the body. He did, however, observe that muscles contract in response to a stimulus from nerves, and he demonstrated experimentally that the arteries carried blood and not air. These observations may possibly have been derived from vivisection, which numerous sources indicate that he practiced.

It is also significant to point out that the Catholic Church did not allow Galen's ideas to be criticised. To question the works of Galen was essentially heresy. He was even called the "Medical Pope" of the Middle Ages. This permitted Galen's erroneous ideas to be perpetuated for approximately 15 centuries. Advancements in the field of anatomy did not occur until the 16th and 17th centuries.

The two internal cerebral veins of Galen unite posteriorly in the region of the pineal body to form the single great cerebral vein of Galen that empties into the straight sinus.

The great cerebral vein of Galen drains blood from the brain into the dural venous sinuses.

ANATOMY DURING
THE MIDDLE AGES

400-1400

The Middle Ages, or Dark Ages, are characterised as an era of intellectual stagnation. Disease was regarded as being of divine origin. It was man's soul and not the human body that was regarded to be important. The outstanding characteristic of the era centered around the acceptance of magic and the influence of the stars on human behavior. Zodiac signs were commonly used to represent various anatomical body parts. Little if any progress was made in the field of anatomy.

In the year 1231, Frederick II decreed that a human body should be dissected at the University of Salerno at least once every five years. Following the death of Frederick in 1250, the dissections were abandoned. The first true university was founded in Bologna, where in 1325 Mondino was given credit for the revival of human dissection. Unfortunately, the practice of human dissection was forgotten after the death of Mondino. Anatomical studies were later revived in France at the University of Montpellier. Permission was granted in 1376 to allow a dissection, on an annual basis, of an executed criminal. There is historical evidence that a few dissections were legalised in other cities in Italy, Spain, and Germany.

It is interesting to note that the anatomists at this time still followed the teachings of Galen and if a dissection revealed a deviation from Galen's teachings, the anatomists concluded that the body was abnormal.

ANATOMY DURING
THE RENAISSANCE

1350-1650

From the very beginning, the advancement of anatomy was influenced by two distinct groups of people. A few physicians and students advocated for dissection, but most individuals opposed dissection. The latter group fought dissection because of their superstitions concerning the dead, their belief in Galen, and the influence of the Church. Neither the teacher nor students touched the cadaver which is a carry over from earlier attitudes.

The influence of artists and their interest in depicting the beauty of the human body on canvas was highly significant in the legalisation of human dissection. The legalisation of human dissection in turn provided an adequate supply of anatomical material for the teaching of anatomy. Leonardo da Vinci (1452-1519) and Michelangelo (1475-1576) were both involved in dissecting as well as painting the human body. It was da Vinci who was the most outstanding artist-anatomist of the Renaissance period. He was a strong advocate for dissecting in order to learn and paint human anatomy.

Andreas Vesalius (1514-1564)

Andreas Vesalius, born in Brussels, is the "founder of human anatomy." He was and still is recognised as the greatest anatomist of all time and was the first anatomist to place his study on a firm foundation of dissection and observation. Vesalius studied under Jacques Sylvius and Johannes Guinterius, both Galenists in doctrine and method.

Both Vesalius and his students stole and personally dissected cadavers. He resented the lecturing and theorising from Galen's text and expressed a

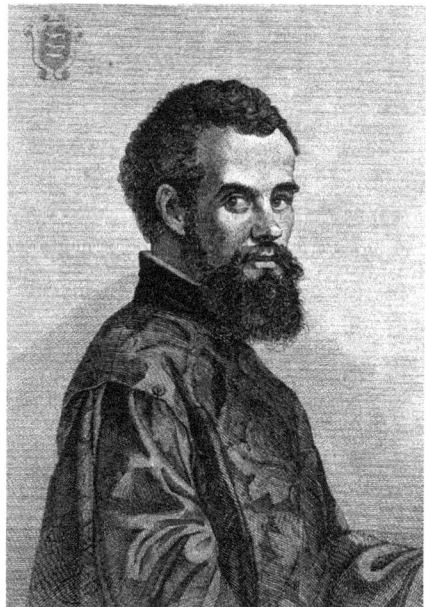

desire to dissect without the use of prosectors whom he considered to be ignorant and uncouth barbers. Vesalius neutralised the authority of Galen and delivered to the field of anatomy a different approach for understanding the human body. He essentially freed anatomical pedagogy from the Galen era by dissecting in person and dispensing with the barber-surgeon, the individual whose duty was to point out the anatomy of the cadaver while the lecturer, at a safe distance, explained it to them. He restructured the longstanding errors and superstitions concerning the human body with beautiful and accurate illustrations from his dissections. Because Vesalius had created the greatest revolution in anatomy and medicine, he was called the "Luther of Anatomy."

Vesalius frequently combed a local cemetery where the bodies of executed criminals were buried, looking for anatomical material. Apparently, Vesalius was very religious and always sought forgiveness prior to the dissection of a cadaver.

He wrote, at the age of 28, the masterpiece of all anatomy textbooks, *De Humani Corporis Fabrica* ("On the Workings of the Human Body"), in which the various human body systems and individual organs were beautifully illustrated and accurately described. Vesalius was introduced to an extraordinary artist named Jan Stephan van Calcar who later painted the anatomical illustrations in the *Fabrica*.

The *Fabrica* is the foundation of modern medicine as a science. This book challenged Galen's teachings and thus caused Vesalius to receive a great deal of scorn from traditional anatomists. Jacques Sylvius, a former mentor, "spoke of Vesalius as a madman, whose pestilential breath poisoned Europe." *De Humani Corporis Fabrica*, published in 1543, revolutionised the science of anatomy and marked the beginning of modern medicine. Sir William Osler even regarded the *Fabrica* as the greatest medical book ever written.

Vesalius appeared in Venice in 1564 and was on his way to the Holy Land. Several stories have been printed concerning the explanation for this journey. The common story was that he apparently obtained permission to perform a post-mortem on a young Spanish nobleman who had died while he was in attendance. During the autopsy and to the horror of the bystanders, Vesalius observed the heart beating. It is highly unlikely that Vesalius with his vast experience with cadaver dissections should have mistaken a living body for a corpse. According to numerous stories, he apparently informed the youth's parents who, along with his enemies, demanded immediate punishment. Apparently, in the inquisition,

Vesalius was given the death sentence. The King of Spain interceded on his behalf with the stipulation that Vesalius make a journey to the Holy Land to seek forgiveness. The available evidence clearly indicates that Vesalius did travel to Jerusalem and was returning to Italy when his ship encountered a storm and sank. It is assumed with some certainty that on his return he fell ill with plague or fever and died in Zante, Greece at the age of fifty on October 15, 1564.

The foresight for the future of anatomy and the evolvement of medicine is all illustrated in the title page of Vesalius's *Fabrica*. There can be no argument that the woodcut should be regarded as one of the finest achievements of art in the sixteenth century. There are numerous symbolisms that reflect Vesalius's vision for anatomical understanding and how this information will be translated into the practice of medicine.

The scene depicts a public dissection conducted by Vesalius, surrounded by his students, fellow physicians, and probably members of the church, dissecting a cadaver with his own hands. This is symbolic of breaking with previous tradition and authority. He has descended from the chair, dispensing with the barber-surgeon demonstrators.

Prior to the time of Vesalius, the anatomy professors did not dissect the body themselves, but relegated this menial task to untrained assistants. Numerous art lovers as well as critics have suggested that the quarreling individuals observed beneath the dissecting table are disgruntled assistants, but it is doubtful that Vesalius intended to depict these men as bickering. Vesalius was probably attempting to illustrate that, as teachers of anatomy, our enthusiasm for teaching anatomy sometimes exceeds our students' enthusiasm for learning. It is obvious that the men sitting beneath the dissecting table have little or no interest in the cadaver or in Vesalius's words of wisdom. One could also assume those students crowding around both Vesalius and the cadaver are focused, energetic, and sincere about learning. Fortunately or unfortunately, most professors can relate to both types of students.

Galen's dependence on small animal anatomy may be symbolised in the dog and monkey shown at the bottom of the painting. Since Vesalius constantly challenged Galen's work, it is therefore highly unlikely that Vesalius would acknowledge Galen in his title page. Various books and numerous speakers have thus depicted the animals as scavengers that eat the cadaver scraps. This concept is totally incorrect, as it is rather doubtful that monkeys or dogs would eat human flesh. Vesalius probably chose to place the animals in the painting for two reasons. First, he wanted to show that dissecting a cadaver permitted one to learn and study anatomical structure. The physiology of blood flow, respiration, digestion, and other functions of the body could not be learned from cadavers alone and, therefore, he was emphasising the use of smaller animals (dogs, cats, monkeys, rats, mice, sheep, etc.) for the additional anatomical data. Secondly, Vesalius was depicting his vision for the study of function or what is currently referred to as physiology. Vesalius is considered to be the "Father of Anatomy," and perhaps physiologists should also refer to him as the "Father of Physiology."

The center of the painting is dominated by a skeleton as he was convinced that the study of anatomy begins with the skeleton. This concept still prevails today and you can find one or several skeletons in most dissection laboratories. Medical students are constantly hammered with the significance of bony landmarks and their relationship to specific soft tissues.

The nude figure clinging to the column on the left is not a local "streaker" who decided he wanted to visit Vesalius and his students. Most would say that the nude is symbolic of surface anatomy. Perhaps the nude is symbolic of much more. The title page of the *Fabrica* symbolises the teaching of anatomy and the entire practice of medicine. It depicts the sincere desire to learn about the human body via human and animal dissections. The nude is symbolic of the patient who disrobes and places his trust and confidence in the judgment of his physician. To experience this relationship between patient (nude) and physician (Vesalius) requires an accurate understanding of the human body which includes anatomical structure and function.

Note the appearance of the amphitheater which provided students a better view of the dissection. Even today, the amphitheater design is present in the departments of anatomy and surgery.

Jan Stephan van Calcar, Vesalius's artist, painted the title page for the *Fabrica*, and some individuals have attempted to identify the artist's self-portrait among the students. A former distinguished student of Vesalius, Harvey Cushing, presumed that the student in the second row to the left of the center and holding an open book to be Jan Stefan van Calcar. Likewise, the elderly bearded man seen looking over the balcony is thought to be the publisher, Johannes Oporinus.

Vesalius's title page of the *Fabrica* is symbolic of all that is important in the dissecting room. Dissection of the human cadaver provides the knowledge and understanding of how the body works. Vesalius envisioned that anatomy would be the basic course and the foundation of the medical student's training. Approximately four hundred years later, thanks to Vesalius and his visions, the dissection of cadavers (anatomy) and the function of the body (physiology) is still taught to all medical students either by regional approaches or by systems.

In summary, the title page in Vesalius's *Fabrica* (1543) is symbolic of the teaching of anatomy and the practice of medicine today.

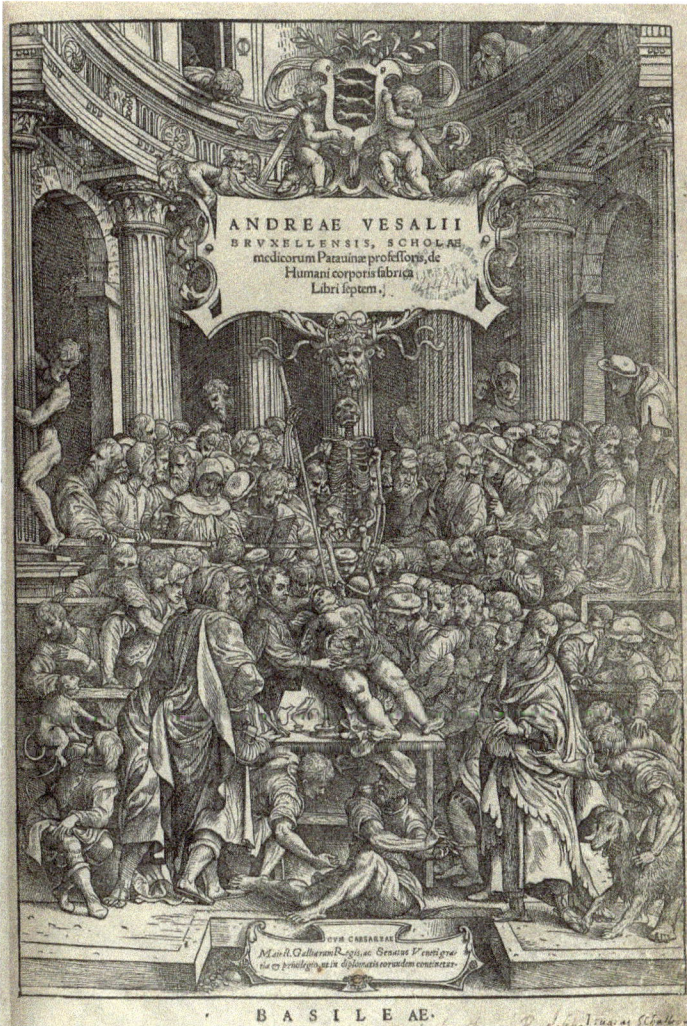

The title page of *De Humani Corporis Fabrica* by Vesalius contains numerous symbols and hidden figures.

THE RISE OF THE RESURRECTIONISTS

1750-1832

Persons who rob bodies from the grave are called "Resurrectionists." During the latter part of the 18th century, the demand for cadavers increased for two reasons: the appointment of full-time professors of anatomy and the rise of private and hospital medical schools.

The "resurrection men" included two distinct groups of individuals. The one group included medical students, physicians, surgeons, and anatomists whose desire for the advancement of science was the motivation; the other was motivated exclusively by money. These human ghouls were low-life thieves.

Providing that the body snatchers – or "sack-'em-up men" – stuck to robbing graves, it was not considered to be a crime even though the activity was disgusting and horrible. Some of the grave robbers, tempted by the money for which a body could be sold, reduced murder to a fine art and made it a lucrative business.

The necessity of having an ample supply of cadavers for the needs of the students in order to prevent the migration of students to rival schools caused the teachers to pay exorbitant prices for the anatomical material. It also forced some of the medical students and teachers to become thieves and ghouls themselves. The increase in demand and the higher prices paid for the cadavers attracted a greater number of vicious and violent individuals to engage in the traffic of cadavers. The teachers were subject to extortion and blackmail by the resurrection men. They held the upper hand over the teachers of anatomy for two reasons: the need for cadavers and the illegality of its source.

Joshua Brooks had created a reputation as one of the best practical anatomists in England. His dealings and sometimes disputes with the London resurrectionists caused him a great deal of notoriety. Badly decomposed bodies were frequently placed in his front yard, causing a fury with the local population. Both his life and his school were saved by the protection of the police.

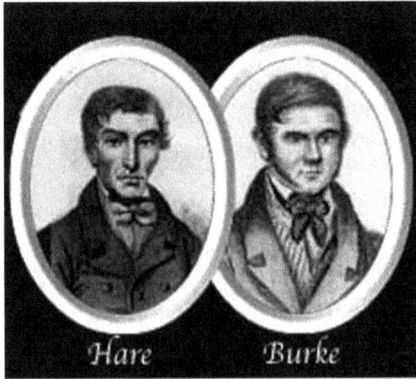

Hare   Burke

The famous Edinburgh case of Burke and Hare began on November 29, 1827, when an elderly man named Donald died at the boarding house owned by William Hare. Donald apparently was in debt to Hare and therefore Hare sought to collect the debt by selling the remains to the local anatomist. Hare discovered an accomplice in William Burke, another of his lodgers. Later the body was transferred to Dr. Knox's dissecting laboratory.

The large sum of money obtained for Donald's body was the motivation for future transactions. Waiting for another death was much too slow and unpredictable. This led to a new and totally unheard of career in crime.

Hare suggested a quicker method of making money, namely, to invite older or drunk individuals to his boarding house where Burke and Hare would kill them. Burke's mistress Helen McDougal along with Hare and his wife worked as a team which allowed the women to lure men from the local taverns to Hare's lodging house where the murders took place. The bodies were later taken to Dr. Knox's anatomical laboratory for dissection.

In less than one year, fifteen additional murders were committed by Burke and Hare and the remains sold to Dr. Knox for dissection. The age or sex of the individual did not matter and consequently the victims included orphans, drunks, widows, and prostitutes. One such case involved a young and beautiful prostitute by the name of Mary Patterson, who was a local and well known streetwalker. Most of the medical students knew Mary and began asking questions when her body turned up in the dissection laboratory. Knox was so impressed with the features of Mary, that he preserved her body for several months in alcohol and invited an artist to sketch it. Robert Louis Stevenson, in his book, *The Body Snatchers*, used Mary as one of his main characters. Several books revolved around the Burke and Hare episodes. Both Charles Dickens' *A Tale of Two Cities* and Thomas Hood's *Mary's Ghost*, were closely associated with the Burke and Hare characters.

Another case involving Burke and Hare revolved around a young mentally impaired individual named James Wilson who was liked and well known. Apparently, Mrs. Hare invited James to the boarding house where Hare killed him and delivered his body to the dissecting laboratory of Dr. Knox. The sudden and mysterious disappearance of James attracted a great deal of attention by the local citizens of Edinburgh.

The last of the Burke and Hare murders involved a woman named Mary Docherty who was killed and stuffed under a pile of straw beneath Burke's bed. Former lodgers, Mr. and Mrs. Gray, while partying with Burke, McDougal, and the Hares, discovered the body and reported it to the authorities. The body was later located in Knox's dissecting laboratory and once it became known that a woman had been murdered for the sale of her body to an Edinburgh anatomist, there were riots and demands for accountability far beyond the limits of Edinburgh.

The career of the murderers lasted for one year ending on Halloween 1828. The trial of Burke and McDougal began on December 24 and ended on Christmas morning. Burke was found guilty of murder and sentenced to be hanged, publicly dissected, and anatomised. McDougal was found not guilty of murder and freed. She later died in Australia. Hare and his wife saved their necks by turning over King's evidence. Mrs. Hare died in Paris. Hare, with the protection of the authorities, was able to leave Scotland and enter England. His identity was discovered by several workmen who promptly threw him into a lime pit which destroyed his eyes. Hare existed as a blind beggar for over forty years.

Dr. Robert Knox, an eloquent and excellent anatomist, who was reputed to be one of the most outstanding anatomical instructors, had his life and reputation wrecked and ruined by his association with Burke and Hare. The Edinburgh townsmen wanted Knox hanged. The courts were unable to prove Knox guilty of any punishable crime other than his association with the notorious grave robbers. Prior to his death, Burke confessed that Dr. Robert Knox was not involved in any of the Edinburgh murders. Burke's confession completely exonerated Dr. Knox. Unfortunately, it was too late to save his reputation, and many of his anatomical contemporaries showed open hostility.

John Hunter, a highly respected anatomist and honored member of the medical profession, was truly a resurrectionist who robbed graves and associated with the scum of the earth. O'Brien, the famous Irish giant (eight feet, four inches tall) was in poor health for several months prior to his death. O'Brien learned that John Hunter was interested in obtaining his skeleton and he therefore took precautions to ensure that his body did not fall into the hands of Hunter. O'Brien paid the undertaker in advance and gave him instructions that his body be placed in a lead coffin and carried to sea and sunk. Apparently, Hunter was able to bribe the undertaker with approximately 500 pounds and thus O'Brien's magnificent skeleton now adorns the Hunterian Museum in the Royal College of Surgeons in London.

The vengeful attitude of the grave robbers occurred not only in England but also in the United States. One of the more famous American grave robbers was known as "Old Cunny," whose ghoulish job required him to supply cadavers to the Ohio Medical College in Cincinnati, Ohio. Upset with some of the medical students who had played a trick on him, he dug up the remains of a small-pox victim and successfully infected a number of the medical class with the horrible disease.

The only known case of an individual having been murdered and sold to an anatomical laboratory in the United State occurred in Baltimore in 1886. A well-known lady by the name of Emily Brown, daughter of a respectable innkeeper, eventually, under the influence of alcohol and drugs, became a streetwalker. She was murdered by a porter who worked at the University of Maryland, and her body was sold to the anatomy department for approximately fifteen dollars. The murderer was apprehended, convicted, and hanged on September 9, 1887.

Students at the now extinct Winchester Medical College, located in Winchester, Virginia, along with the professor of anatomy frequently searched the local cemeteries for anatomical material. A number of the medical students were attracted to Harper's Ferry in October of 1859, at the time John Brown - the abolitionist - was there attacking the federal arsenal. The students traveled by train from Winchester and as they departed the train, they discovered a dead body, and naturally looking for sources of anatomical material, immediately packed the body and shipped it back to the medical college in Winchester. They discovered papers on the body that indicated it was Owen Brown the son of John Brown. The body was dissected and the remains were returned much later to Winchester.

A body snatching episode of huge magnitude occurred in Ohio in 1878. U.S. Senator John Scott Harrison died and was buried. He was the son of William Henry Harrison, who served as President of the United States for one month in 1841, and the father of Benjamin Harrison who became President in 1888. It was later accidentally discovered that the body of John Scott Harrison was in the process of being dissected in the Medical College of Ohio. Public sentiment exploded and the news media demanded reprisal against not only the grave robbers but also the entire field of medicine and anatomy.

The passage of the Warburton Anatomy Act in 1832 ended the vocation of body snatching, which had long been regarded as a despicable but necessary evil. Prior to the above mentioned dates, the only legalised source of cadavers resulted from the execution of criminals.

MODERN ANATOMY

1900-2011

Most if not all medical students are familiar with *Gray's Anatomy*, originally published by the English surgeon Sir Henry Gray in 1858. Since then *Gray's Anatomy* has had numerous authors and has evolved into the current fortieth edition in Great Britain and the thirtieth edition in the United States.

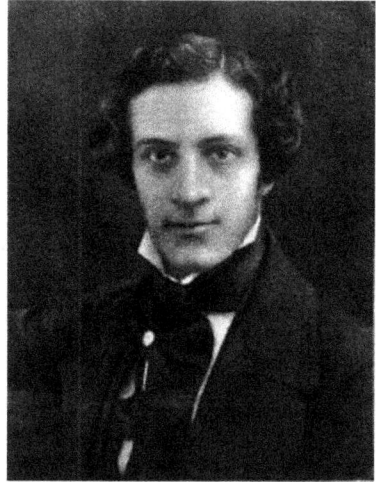

There is an interesting fact concerning the fifth American editor, Edward Spitzka, who became interested in the differences between criminal brains and those of so called normal brains. He attended many electrocutions, recording his observations of the effect of electrical death on the human brain. He also removed the brains immediately after death. It was rumored that his keen interest in the brains of criminals and his regular attendance at all electrocutions was noted by the members of the criminal underworld. Many of the local thugs became furious and threatened to kill Spizka if he were to remove the brain of any member of their gang. These life and death threats apparently caused Spizka to become paranoid as he was in constant fear for his life. He lectured at Jefferson Medical College, where on one occasion he entered the lecture room, drew six shooters from each side of his belt, checked behind the doors, examined all nooks and corners of the room with both guns in hand, proceeded to the lecture podium, placed the guns on the desk, and then proceeded to deliver his lecture.

Because of the current streamlined medical curricula, *Gray's Anatomy*, still regarded as the "Anatomical Bible" is rarely recommended as the textbook, as it contains more anatomical information than is considered necessary for medical students. Most of the current textbooks of anatomy include only the essentials.

Cadaver dissections, despite reduction in allocated time, continue to consume a significant portion of the first-year medical curriculum. Cadavers are obtained through donations and unclaimed bodies. Neither medical students nor the professors of anatomy are involved in the procurement of bodies for the anatomical laboratories.

Because of the limited time allocated for anatomy, the numerous anatomists whose names – or eponyms – have been attached to specific anatomical nomenclature, have disappeared from the instruction of anatomy. Unfortunately, without eponyms, the human aspect of medical history is lost.

References

Ball, James Moore. *The Sack Em-Up Men*. Edinburgh. 1928
Dobson, Jessie. *Anatomical Eponyms*. Edinburgh. 1962
Dorland's *Illustrated Medical Dictionary*. Philadelphia. 1981
Goss, Charles M. *Henry Gray and his Anatomy*. Philadelphia. 1959
Lassek, A.M. *Human Dissection*. Springfield. 1957
Lind, L.R. *The Epitome of Andreas Vesalius*. Cambridge. 1949
Moore, Wendy. *The Knife Man*. New York. 2005

INTEGUMENTARY SYSTEM

Michael Stanley Clive Birbeck
1925-2005

Birbeck was an electron microscopist at the Chester Beatty Cancer Research Institute in London. He discovered Birbeck granules, which are found within Langerhans cells in the epidermis of the skin. They are cytoplasmic organelles shaped like a tennis racket with a central linear density and a striated appearance.

Sir Astley Cooper
1768-1841

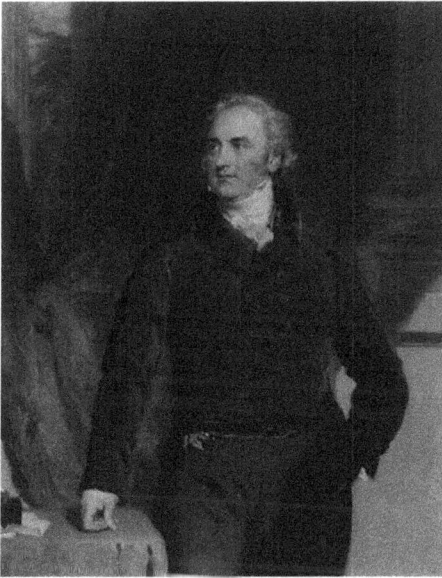

Sir Cooper was one of the most famous surgeon-anatomists of that particular era. The resurrectionists, also known as body snatchers, were extremely active from 1800 to 1832, and it was also the time that Sir Cooper performed most of his anatomical dissections. Grave robbing, which was at its peak, provided Sir Cooper with the anatomical material necessary to run his dissection laboratory. In spite of publicly describing the body snatchers as "rascals and the lowest dregs of society," he was fully committed to, and totally dependent upon, the grave robber for his dissecting material. Alliances between eminent anatomists and the most despicable grave robbers were made imperative. The breast is supported by the suspensory ligaments of Cooper, which are strong fibrous processes that penetrate the breast tissue, connecting the dermis of the skin to the deep layer of the superficial fascia. Cooper's ligament is also another name for the pectineal ligament, which is a strong fibrous band that extends from the lacunar ligament along the pectineal line of the pubis.

Thomas Henry Huxley
1825-1895

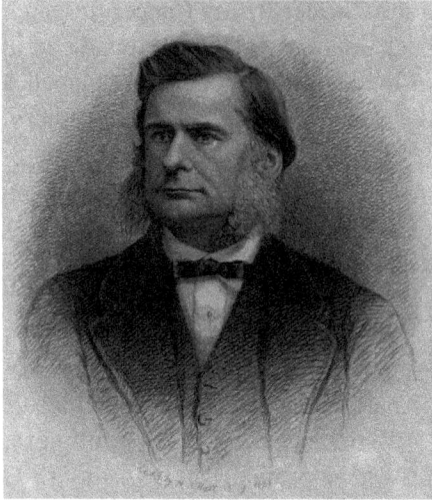

Henry Huxley was an English surgeon well known for his advocacy of Charles Darwin. He wrote a paper as a 19-year-old medical student describing the internal root sheath of the hair follicle, which is composed of Henle's layer, Huxley's layer, and the cuticle.

Huxley's layer is a component of the hair follicle.

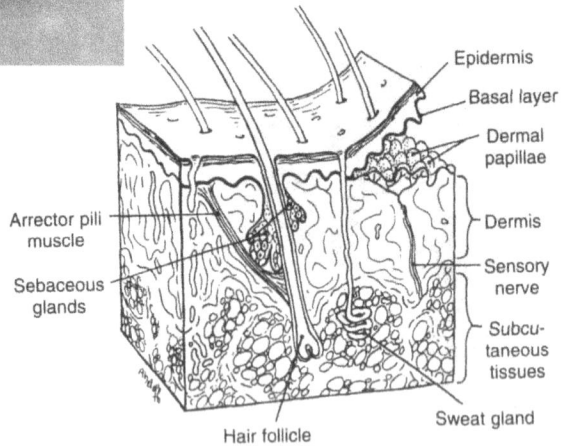

Wilhelm Krause
1833-1909

Wilhelm Krause was an anatomist and histologist whose greatest contribution was associated with acino-tubular glands which had been previously discovered by his father Karl Krause. Krause's glands refer to the conjunctival glands that were previously described by his father. Krause's end bulbs are cold and pressure receptors in the deep portion of the dermis.

Karl Langer
1819-1887

Karl Langer was an anatomist who first described cleavage lines of the skin, known as Langer's lines, which were related to the disposition of subcutaneous fibrous tissue.

Marcello Malpighi
1628-1694

Marcello Malpighi first demonstrated the structure and function of the lung. He is considered by many to be the founder of microscopic anatomy, also known as histology. His descriptions on skin were exceedingly good, and he likewise contributed a great deal to our knowledge of the spleen. The two deepest layers of the epidermis (stratum basale and stratum spinosum) are collectively referred to as the Malpighian layer and are an area of high mitotic activity. The capsule of the spleen is commonly referred to as Malpighi's capsule, and the splenic corpuscles (Malpighi's corpuscles) are likewise associated with the investigator.

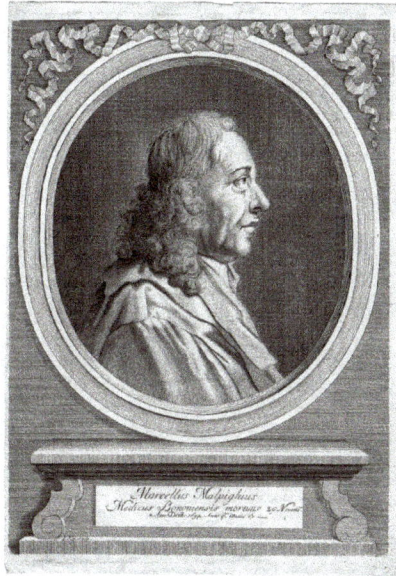

Marcellus Malpighius Medicus Bononiensis

The epidermis, the deepest layer of which is the Malpighian layer, occupies most of this micrograph. The "outside world" is at the upper left, and the dermis, with its fingerlike projections, is at the lower right.

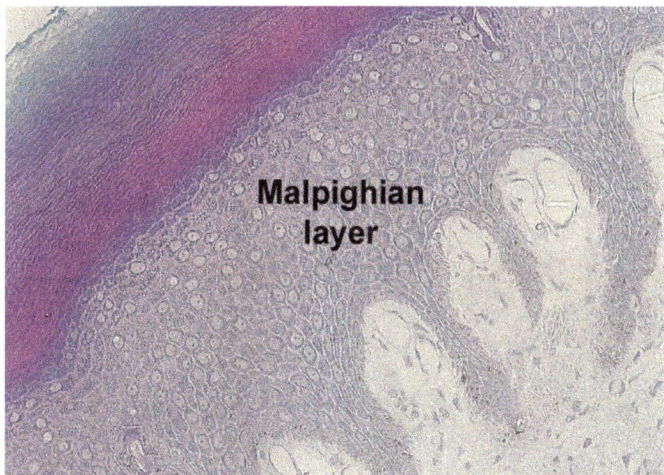

Malpighian layer

James Spence
1812-1882

James Spence, Professor of Surgery at the University of Edinburgh, was the first to describe a lateral process of mammary tissue that extends from the mammary gland to the axillary region and is referred to as the axillary tail of Spence.

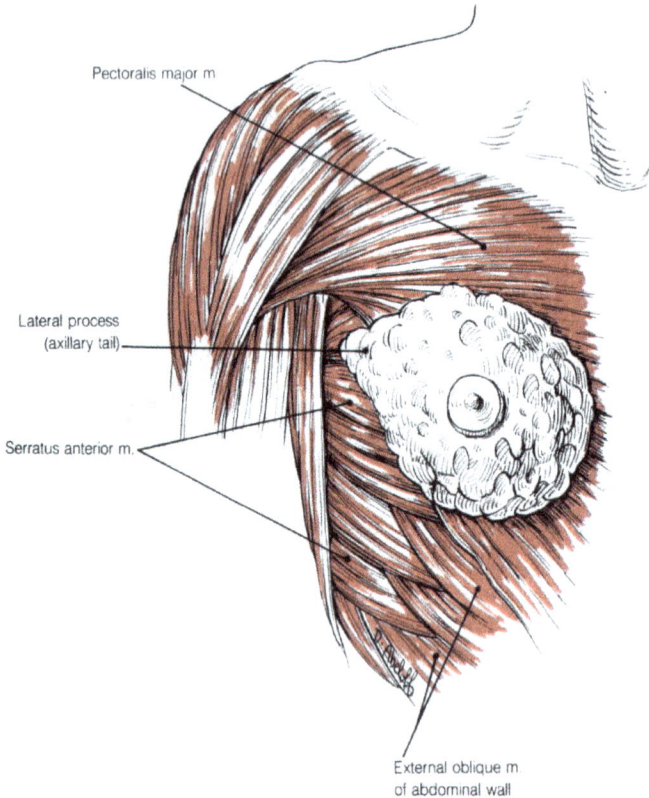

Pectoralis major m

Lateral process
(axillary tail)

Serratus anterior m.

External oblique m
of abdominal wall

The lateral process of the breast, also known as the axillary tail of Spence, is seen at the periphery of the breast near the axilla, or armpit.

MUSCULOSKELETAL SYSTEM

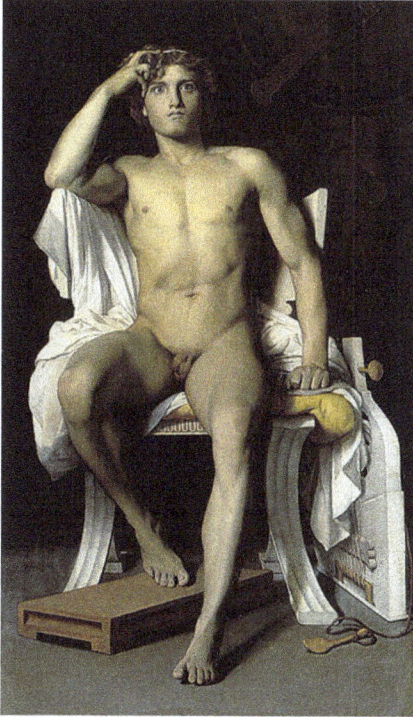

Achilles

Achilles was a Greek hero of the Trojan War. Legend says that his body was invulnerable except for his heel, by which his mother held him as a baby as she dipped him in the river Styx to render him immortal. He ultimately died due to a poisoned arrow shot into his heel. Thus the term "Achilles' heel" has come to refer to a person's main weakness. The tendo calcaneus is known as the Achilles tendon.

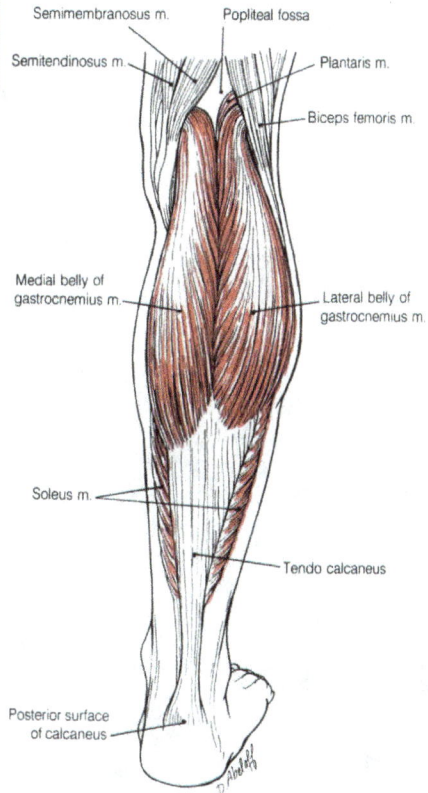

The tendo calcaneus is more commonly known as the Achilles tendon.

Semimembranosus m.
Popliteal fossa
Semitendinosus m.
Plantaris m.
Biceps femoris m.
Medial belly of gastrocnemius m.
Lateral belly of gastrocnemius m.
Soleus m.
Tendo calcaneus
Posterior surface of calcaneus

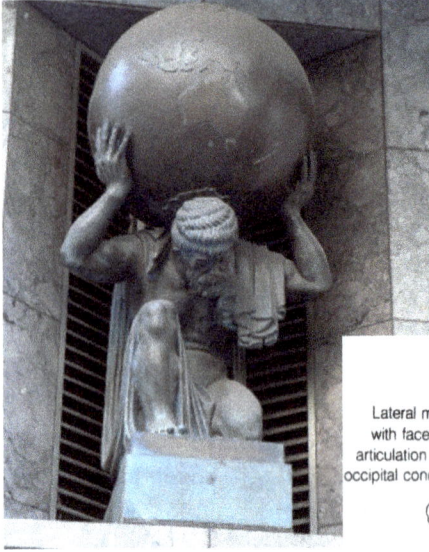

The first cervical vertebra, or atlas, holds the head just as Atlas held the world.

Atlas

Atlas, a character from Greek mythology, was punished by Zeus and made to bear the weight of the heavens on his back. The first cervical vertebra, the atlas, articulates with the occipital condyles of the occipital bone of the skull above.

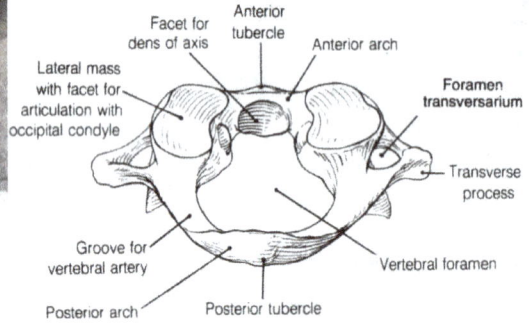

Henry Jacob Bigelow
1818-1890

Bigelow served as Professor of Surgery in the medical school of Harvard University in Boston, Massachusetts. He was given credit for the discovery of the iliofemoral ligament which is described as the "Y"-shaped ligament of the hip joint.

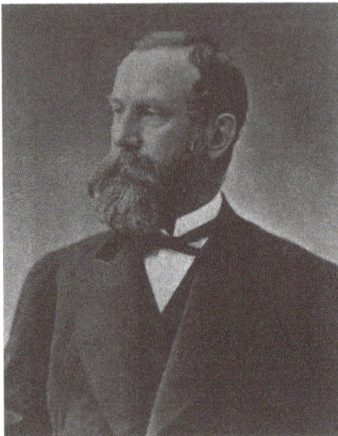

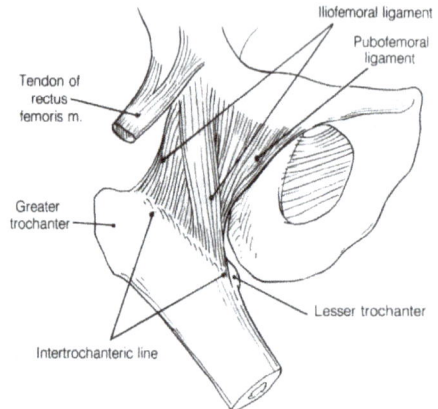

The iliofemoral ligament is often still called the ligament of Bigelow.

Allan Burns
1781-1813

Burns, an anatomist, served as a lecturer in Glasgow, Scotland, at a private school run by his brother John. Burns was given credit for describing the falciform ligament of the fascia lata at the saphenous opening in the thigh which is currently referred to as Burns's ligament. His name is most notably associated with the fascial space located at the jugular notch (Burns's space); this region is known as an erogenous zone as well as a target in the martial arts. Burns died from a dissecting wound.

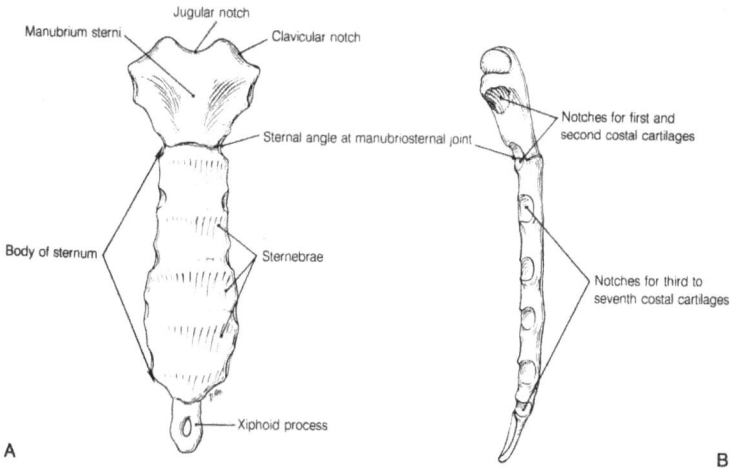

The jugular notch, also known as Burns's space, has been referenced in numerous movies.

Peter Camper
1722-1789

Camper, a Dutchman, was not only a physician and anatomist but also a paleontologist, anthropologist and artist. Interested in comparative mammalian anatomy, he discovered that the bones of birds were hollow. Camper was one of the greatest teachers of the century. The superficial fatty layer of the superficial fascia of the abdomen is commonly referred to as Camper's fascia.

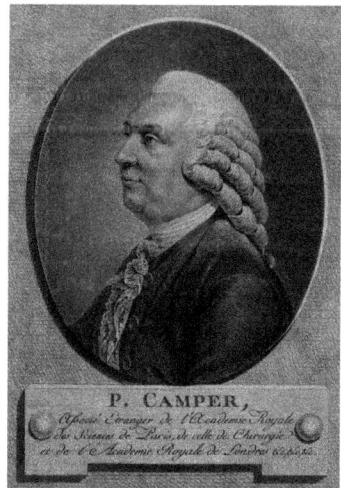

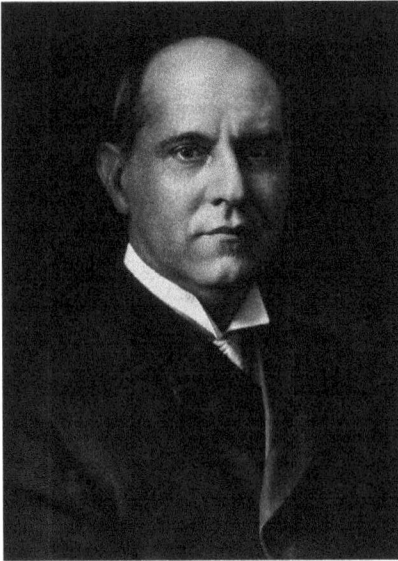

Charles Chassaignac
1805-1879

Chassaignac was a surgeon who first recognised the significance of the tubercle of the 6th cervical vertebra. Numerous anatomical relationships can be associated with Chassaignac's tubercle. It is located at the level of the entrance of the vertebral artery into the vertebral canal and is hence referred to as the carotid tubercle. The carotid pulse can easily be obtained by pressing the carotid artery against this tubercle. Chassaignac's tubercle is also a useful anatomical landmark when seeking the junction of the pharynx and the esophagus, especially the location of a pharyngoesophageal fistula. Chassaignac's space is commonly referred to as the retromammary space which is located between the pectoralis major and the mammary gland.

Jules Germain Cloquet
1790-1883

Jules Cloquet was a French anatomist and surgeon whose brother Hippolyte studied the nasopalatine nerve in the incisive canal. Jules Cloquet is given credit for the discovery of the vestigium processus vaginalis which is referred to as Cloquet's Ligament. Furthermore, he is associated with Cloquet's node, a prominent lymph node in the superior aspect of the thigh.

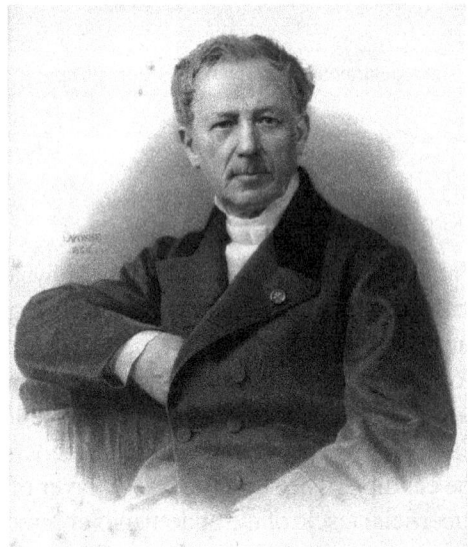

Abraham Colles
1773-1843

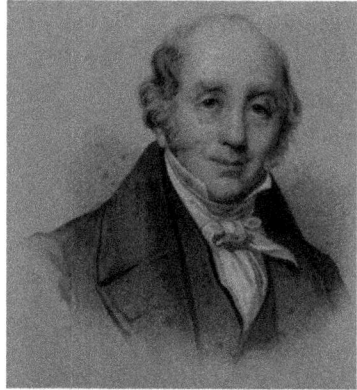

Colles was born in Ireland but studied both in Ireland and Scotland. After working with Sir Astley Cooper in London, he was Professor of Anatomy and Surgery in Ireland. The deep layer of the superficial fascia of the perineum is commonly referred to as Colles's fascia.

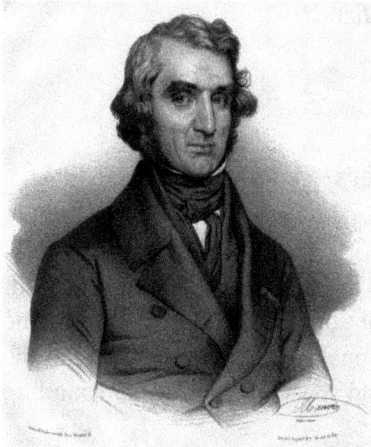

Pierre Nicolas Gerdy
1797-1856

Gerdy, a French surgeon, anatomist, physiologist and pathologist, was the first to describe the suspensory ligament of the axilla. Gerdy's tubercle is a projection on the lateral aspect of the tibia where the iltiotibial band of the fascia lata inserts.

Manuel Louise Antonio don Gimbernat
1734-1816

Gimbernat, a surgeon and anatomist in Barcelona, was director of the Royal College of Surgeons in Spain and a surgeon to King Carlos III. Gimbernat attended William Hunter's Lectures and demonstrated to Hunter a procedure for the identification of the lacunar ligament which was later referred to as Gimbernat's Ligament. It is essentially the extension of the inguinal ligament to the pectineal line of the pubis, forming part of the femoral ring as well as the floor of the inguinal canal.

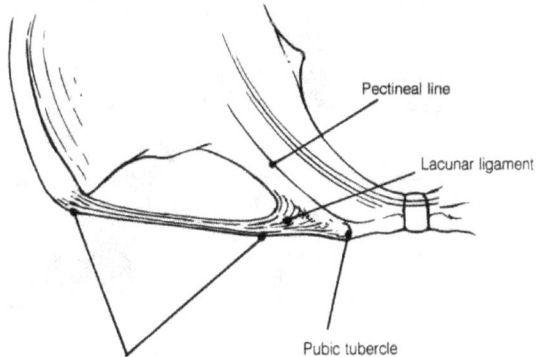

Students are taught to palpate the lacunar ligament, or Gimbernat's ligament, as it marks the edge of the "empty space" medial to the femoral vein.

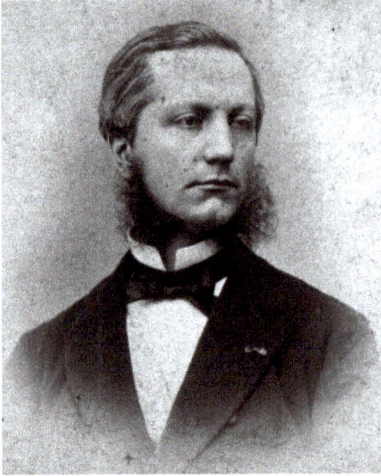

Jean Casimir Felix Guyon
1831-1920

Guyon was a French professor of medicine and pathology. He is affiliated with Guyon's canal, which is also known as the ulnar canal or ulnar tunnel. It is a space in the wrist between the hamate bone and the pisiform bone through which the ulnar nerve and ulnar artery travel from the arm into the hand.

Clopton Havers
1657-1702

Havers, whose birth year is occasionally noted as 1655, was educated at Utrecht in the Netherlands but was a physician in London, England. A Fellow of the Royal Society, he was Gale Lecturer at Surgeons' Hall. Havers was one of the first to describe the Haversian canals as central spaces within the surrounding lamellae of compact bone.

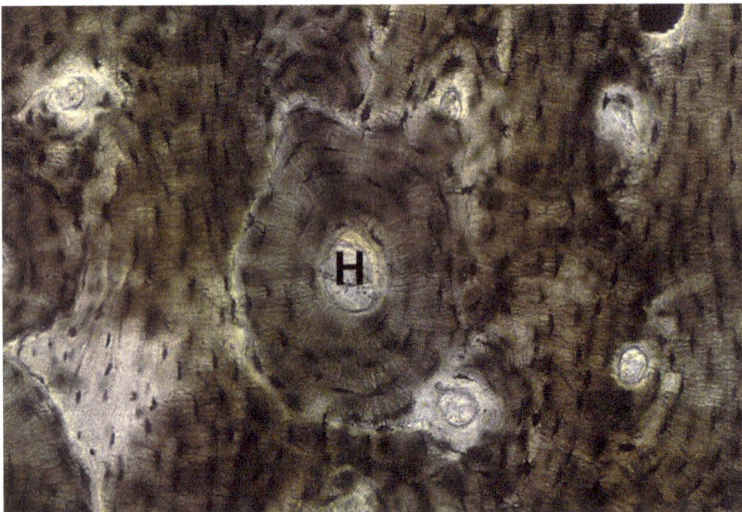

Haversian canals (H) transmit nerves and blood vessels in the osteons of bone.

Franz Kaspar Hesselbach
1759-1816

Hesselbach was a German surgeon and topographical anatomist in Heidelberg and Wurzburg. He is given credit for providing the early description of the cribriform fascia, which is referred to as Hesselbach's fascia, and the interfoveolar ligament, which is also called Hesselbach's ligament. The inguinal triangle bounded by the inferior epigastric artery, the lateral margin of the rectus abdominis muscle, and the inguinal ligament is referred to as Hesselbach's triangle.

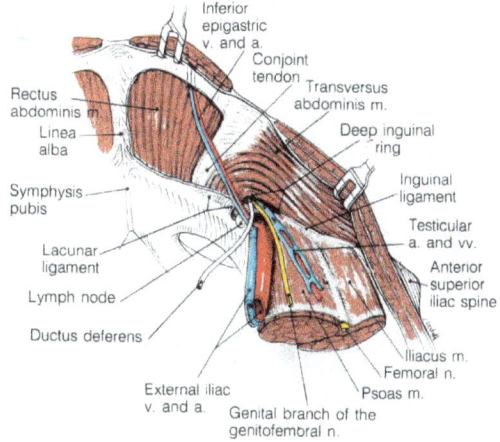

Hesselbach's triangle is bounded by the inferior epigastric artery, rectus abdominis, and inguinal ligament.

John Howship
1781-1841

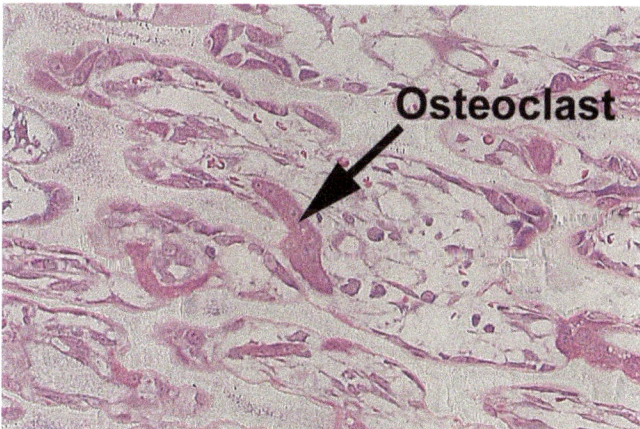

The osteoclast, the pink oblong cell at the arrow, resides in a small pocket of space known as Howship's lacuna.

Howship was an English surgeon who studied pathology of bone because he himself suffered from osteomyelitis. He described the absorption spaces in diseased bone, later referred to as Howship's foveolae, lacunae, or pits. In normal bone, Howship's lacunae are resorption pits where osteoclasts, cells that break down bone, are located.

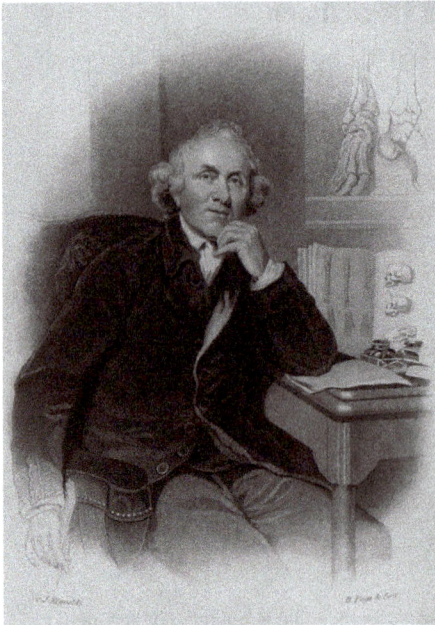

John Hunter
1728-1793

John Hunter, born in Scotland from humble circumstances, rose to become the most famous anatomist and surgeon of the eighteenth century. He performed countless human dissections in the laboratory of his brother, William Hunter. His need for human corpses involved him with the common grave robbers who were known as the body snatchers. He paid huge sums of money for stolen cadavers and was intimately involved in the stealing of the corpse of the famous "Irish Giant." John Hunter was determined to move surgery from the "snake and oil" profession to a more scientific level of modern medicine. Using the knowledge he gained from human dissections, Hunter rejected medieval traditions and pioneered a revolution in surgery founded on scientific experiments. He spent most of his career in London where he was known as an excellent dissector, surgical pioneer, innovative researcher, and passionate educator. Among his patients were Benjamin Franklin and Lord Byron, to name but a few. His scientific successes included tooth transplants, description of the lymphatic system, and study of sexually transmitted diseases, among others. He also developed a unique museum of anatomical specimens, both human and animal. Today he is often regarded as the "Father of Modern Surgery."

An embryonic connection between the testis and the scrotum is referred to as the gubernaculum testis or Hunter's gubernaculum. The subsartorial canal, or adductor canal, conducts the femoral vessels through the middle one-third of the thigh and is commonly referred to as Hunter's canal.

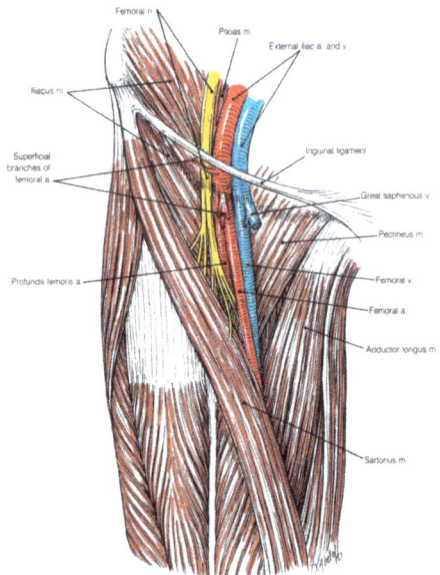

Underneath the sartorius muscle is Hunter's canal, a tunnel containing the femoral vessels.

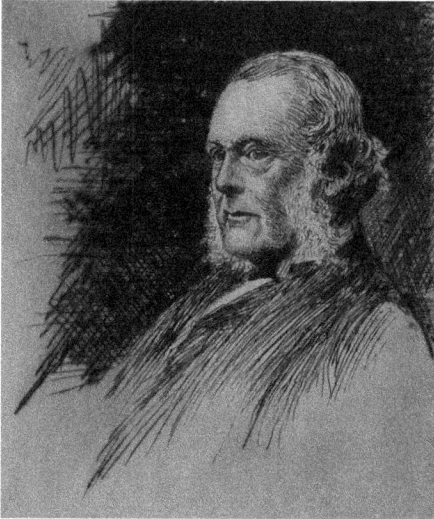

Lord Joseph Lister
1827-1912

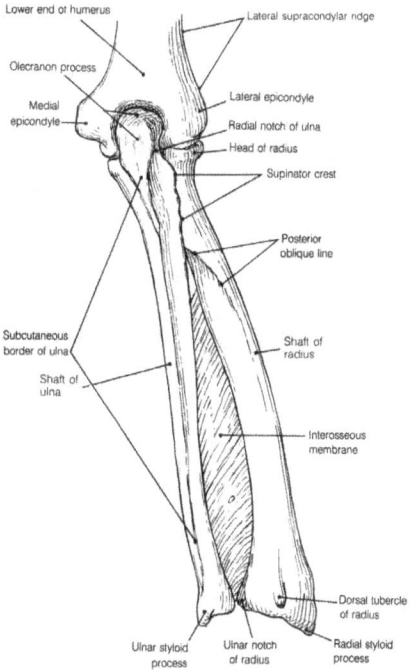

The dorsal tubercle of the radius is often referred to as Lister's tubercle.

Lister, born and educated in London, England, went to Edinburgh, Scotland, where he worked with Syme, whose daughter he married. He then served as Professor of Surgery in Glasgow, Scotland, but returned to Edinburgh where he replaced the resigning Syme as Professor of Surgery. He then returned to London where he served as Professor of Clinical Surgery at King's College. In 1895, he received the Albert Medal of the Royal Society of Arts in recognition of his use of antiseptic methods in surgery.

The prominence located on the dorsal surface of the distal end of the radius adjacent to the depression for the tendon of the extensor pollicis longus is referred to as Lister's tubercle.

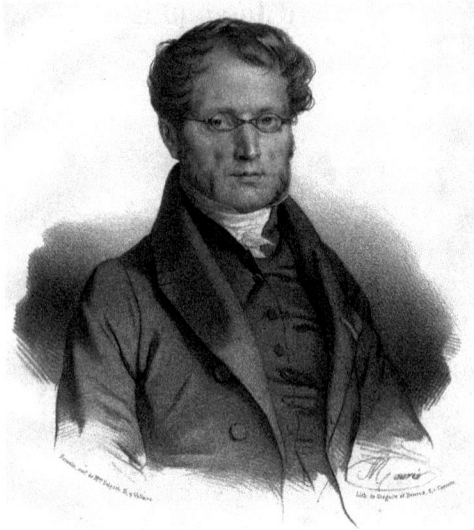

Pierre Charles Alexandre Louis
1787-1872

Louis was a French physician who specialised in tuberculosis. He was the first to acknowledge the angle formed by the manubrium and the body of the sternum which is currently identified as the sternal angle or angle of Louis.

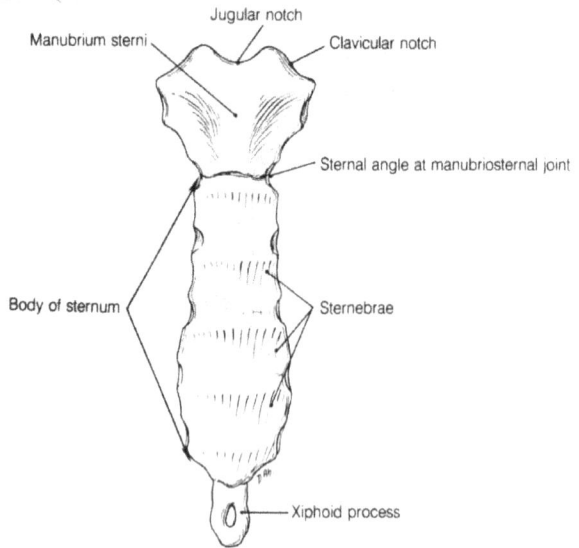

The sternal angle is more often called the angle of Louis and is an important landmark for locating the second rib and second intercostal space.

Jugular notch

Manubrium sterni

Clavicular notch

Sternal angle at manubriosternal joint

Body of sternum

Sternebrae

Xiphoid process

Anton Nuck
1650-1692

Nuck was a Dutchman who was Professor of Anatomy and Medicine in Leyden. The canal of Nuck is an abnormal patent processus vaginalis extending into the labia majora of females.

Jean Louis Petit
1664-1741

Jean Louis Petit, not to be confused with three others bearing the same name, lived in Paris where he was a surgeon and anatomist. At the age of 7, he studied anatomy under Du Littre. He dissected and attended lectures at the age of 12 and was 16 when he became Surgeon to La Charite Hospital.

He defined the triangle located between the crest of the ilium and the margins of the external oblique and latissimus dorsi muscles which is referred to as the lumbar triangle or Petit's triangle.

Francois Poupart
1661-1708

The inguinal ligament used to be commonly referred to as Poupart's ligament.

Poupart was a French surgeon and naturalist who studied not only vertebrate anatomy but also invertebrate anatomy of locusts, worms, leeches, and slugs. Poupart described the inguinal ligament which had been previously described by Falloppius in 1584. The inguinal ligament, also known as Poupart's ligament, is the folded inferior border of the aponeurosis of the external abdominal oblique muscle.

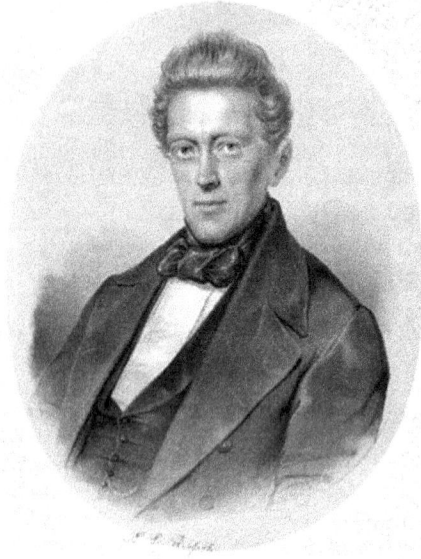

Karl Bogislaus Reichert
1811-1883

Reichert was born in Rastenburg, which was then located in the German province of East Prussia but which is now located in Poland. The German embryologist and comparative anatomist was Professor of Human and Comparative Anatomy in several European cities, including Dorpat, Breslau, and Berlin, where he died. Reichert first described the cartilage of the second branchial arch which is referred to as Reichert's cartilage.

Antonio Scarpa
1747-1832

Scarpa was an Italian anatomist and surgeon who studied at Bologna and later became Professor of Surgery in Modena. His name is recognised for his work in several different areas. He was the first to describe the femoral triangle which includes the subfascial space of the upper one-third of the thigh. The triangle is bounded above by the inguinal ligament, laterally by the medial border of the sartorius muscle, and medially by the medial border of adductor longus muscle. The femoral triangle is called Scarpa's triangle. The ganglion on the vestibular nerve, which is located in the internal auditory meatus, is referred to as Scarpa's ganglion. Most notably, the deep membranous, fibrous, layer of the superficial fascia of the abdominal wall is called Scarpa's fascia.

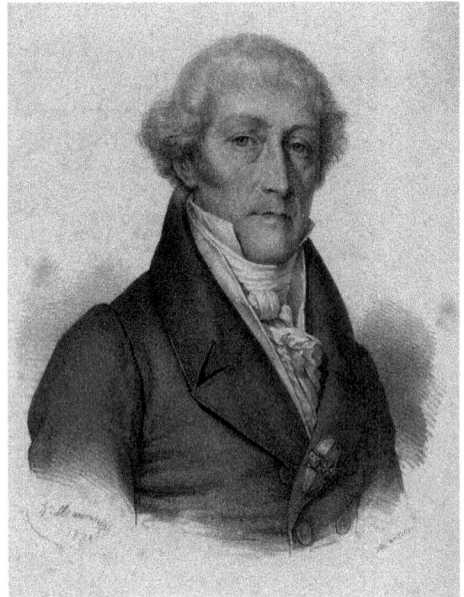

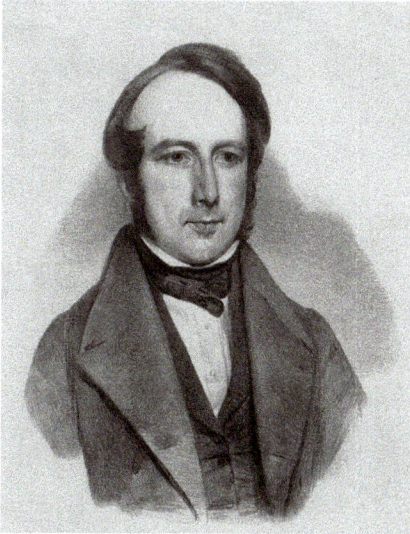

William Sharpey
1802-1880

Sharpey was born in Scotland and studied at University College in London. He served as Professor of Anatomy first in Edinburgh and later in London at University College. He was one of the first to identify and describe the fibers located between the periosteum and the bone. These fibers were referred to as Sharpey's fibers.

Edward Warren Hine Shenton
1872-1955

Shenton, an English radiologist, described a curved line that is formed by the obturator foramen and is seen in the radiograph of the normal hip joint. It is referred to as Shenton's line.

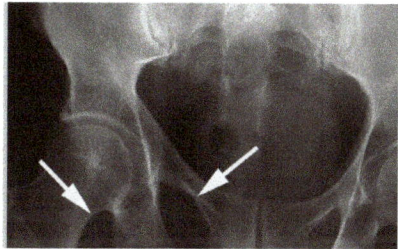

The white arrows delineate Shenton's line.

Alfred Wilhelm Volkmann
1800-1877

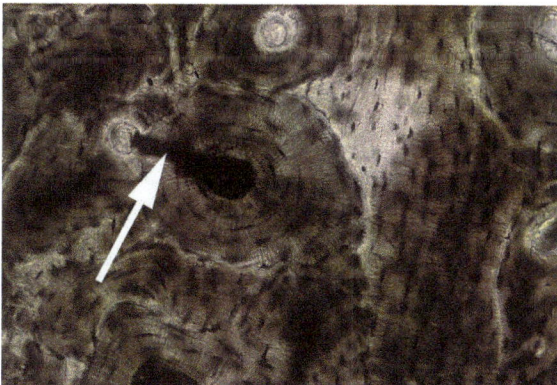

Volkmann, a German professor of physiology and anatomy, was the first man to describe canals in bone that carried blood vessels from the periosteum. These canals were identified as Volkmann's canals.

Volkmann's canal, seen at the white arrow, transmits blood vessels from the periosteum to more internal regions within bone.

NERVOUS SYSTEM

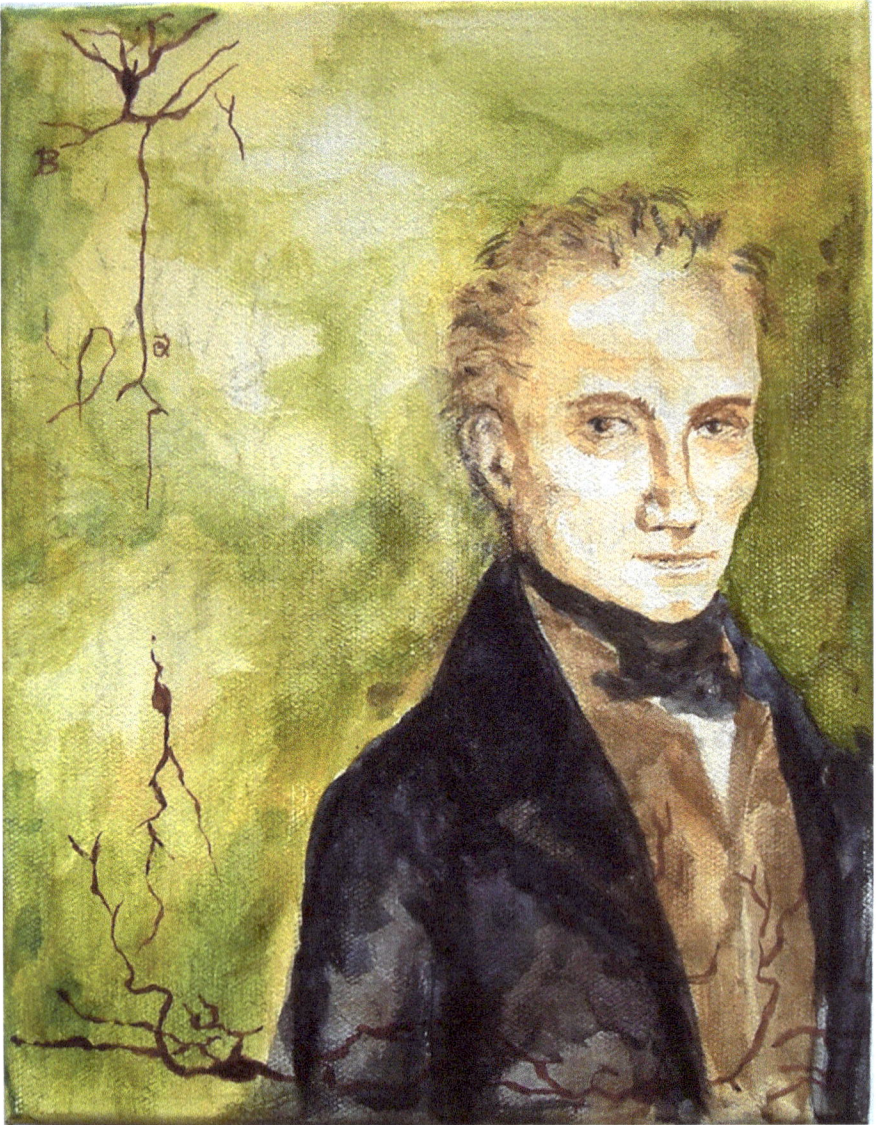

Johannes Evangelista Purkinje
Taken from *The Alphabet of Anatomical Eponyms* ©Meredith Browne
http://meredithbrowne.weebly.com/alphabet-of-anatomical-eponyms.html

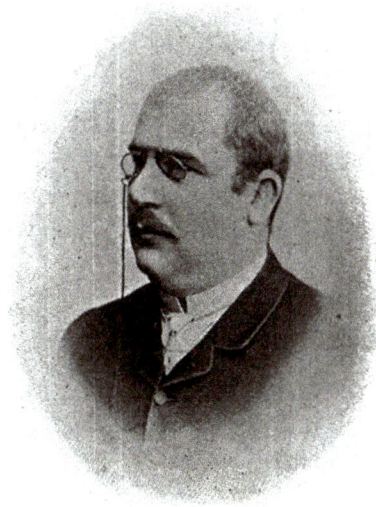

Albert Adamkiewicz
1850-1921

Adamkiewicz was a Polish pathologist who was given credit for the discovery of crescent-shaped cells located beneath the neurilemma of medullated nerve fibers. These cells are referred to as Adamkiewicz's demilunes. The artery of Adamkiewicz is the largest anterior segmental medullary artery supplying the spinal cord. It arises from a left posterior intercostal artery, which branches from the aorta, and supplies the lower two thirds of the spinal cord via the anterior spinal artery.

Friedrich Arnold
1803-1890

Arnold, a German, was a professor of anatomy in Zurich, Freiburg, Tubingen, and Heidelberg. Arnold's name is associated with several anatomical structures. The otic ganglion associated with the mandibular division of the trigeminal nerve is called Arnold's Ganglion, and the auricular branch of the vagus nerve is referred to as Arnold's nerve.

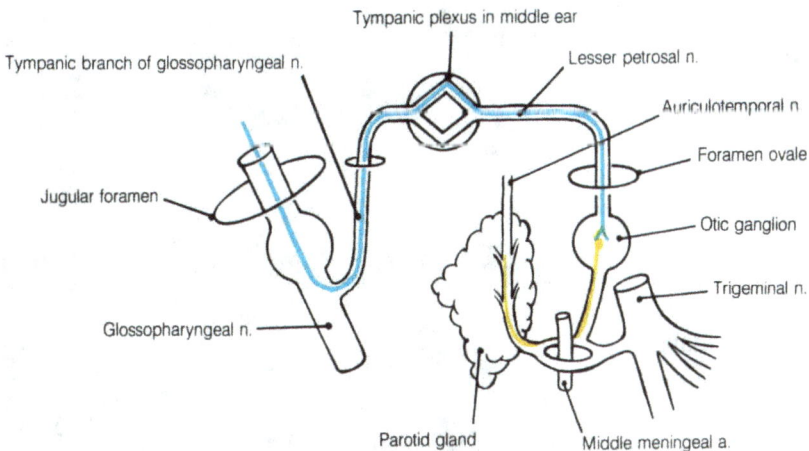

The otic ganglion, or Arnold's ganglion, contains synapses of parasympathetic neurons of the glossopharyngeal nerve.

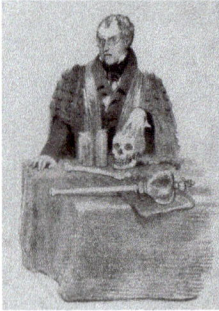

Sir Charles Bell
1774-1842

Sir Charles Bell, whose brother John Bell was a surgeon and anatomist, was a Scottish surgeon and neuroscientist. In addition to running a school of anatomy in Edinburgh, he was also a professor of surgery. Bell was best known for his work on the nervous system. The long thoracic nerve, which innervates the serratus anterior muscle, is commonly called the long thoracic nerve of Bell.

The long thoracic nerve of Bell is derived from spinal nerves C5, C6, and C7 of the brachial plexus.

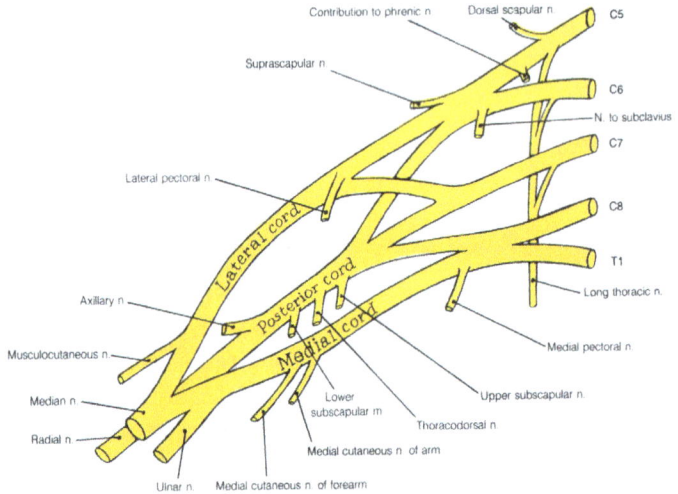

Vladimir Aleksandrovich Betz
1834-1894

Betz was a professor of anatomy in Kiev, Ukraine. He was the first to describe the large pyramidal cells of the motor cortex of the brain. These cells are now commonly referred to as Betz cells.

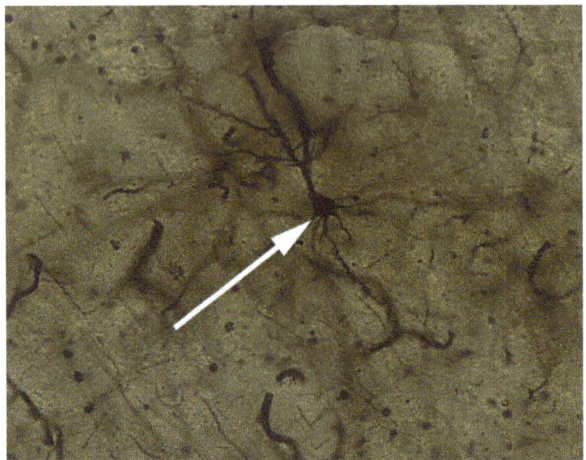

A Betz cell is seen at the tip of the white arrow. Located in the cortex of the brain, these cells have pyramidal cell bodies with branching dendrites.

Pierre Paul Broca
1824-1880

Broca was a surgeon, anatomist, and anthropologist in Paris, France. The so-called "speech area," located in the inferior frontal gyrus of the left cerebral hemisphere of the brain, is commonly called Broca's convolution.

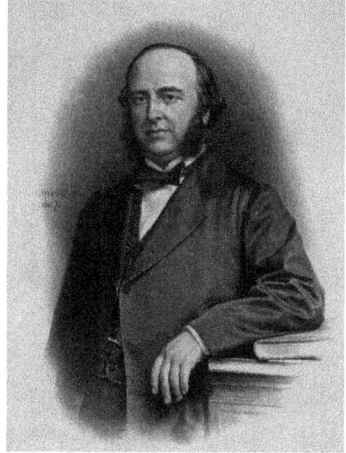

Korbinian Brodmann
1868-1918

Brodmann worked in psychiatric clinics in Germany, was superintendent of the Anatomical Laboratory in Tubingen, and was ultimately a professor. Approximately fifty-two cortical areas of the cerebral hemispheres associated with specific functions are referred to as Brodmann's areas.

Santiago Ramony Cajal
1852-1934

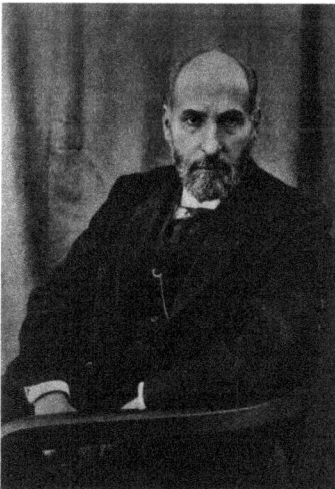

Cajal was a Spanish physician who served as a professor of anatomy, histology and morbid anatomy (now known as anatomical pathology). He is most well known, however, as a neuroscientist. In 1906, he shared the Nobel Prize in Physiology or Medicine with Camillo Golgi for the study of neurons in the central nervous system. The horizontally-oriented multipolar neurons of the cerebral cortex are commonly referred to as Cajal's cells. He is also associated with the interstitial cells of Cajal in the wall of the intestine; these cells serve as pacemaker cells for peristalsis.

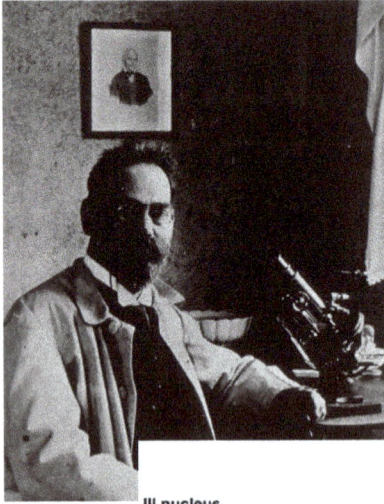

Ludwig Edinger
1855-1918

Edinger was an anatomist and neurologist in Germany. The preganglionic parasympathetic cell bodies of the oculomotor nerve, located in the mesencephalon, are referred to as the Edinger-Westphal nucleus.

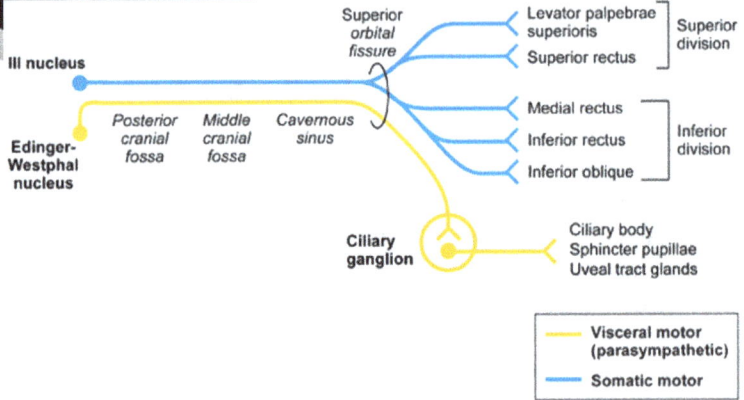

The Edinger-Westphal nucleus in the brainstem is the origin of parasympathetic neurons of the oculomotor nerve.

Wilhelm Heinrich Erb
1840-1921

Erb was a German neurologist. A traumatic lesion of the upper brachial plexus, specifically the fifth and sixth spinal nerves, results in a paralysis known as Erb-Duchenne palsy. Erb's point is a location in the lateral aspect of the neck where several nerves converge at one point.

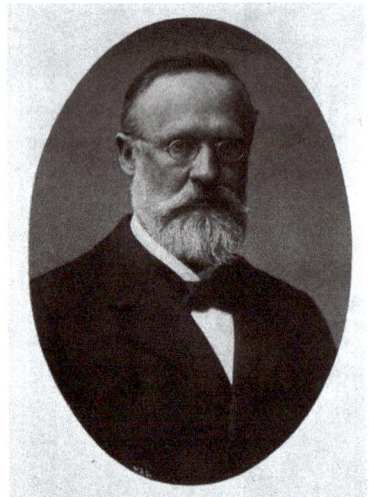

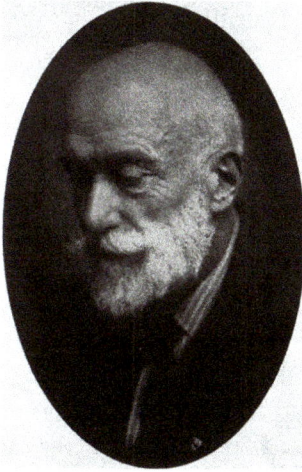

August Forel
1848-1931

Forel was an anatomist and neurologist in Switzerland. The ventral tegmental decussation located between the red nuclei of the mesencephalon of the brain is commonly referred to as Forel's decussation.

Johann Laurentius Gasser
18th Century

Gasser, an Austrian, lived in the 18th century, although the dates of his birth and death are not known. He was a professor of anatomy in Vienna. The trigeminal (semilunar) ganglion, a location of sensory nerve cell bodies of the trigeminal nerve, is also referred to as the Gasserian ganglion. The ganglion was named after him and not by him.

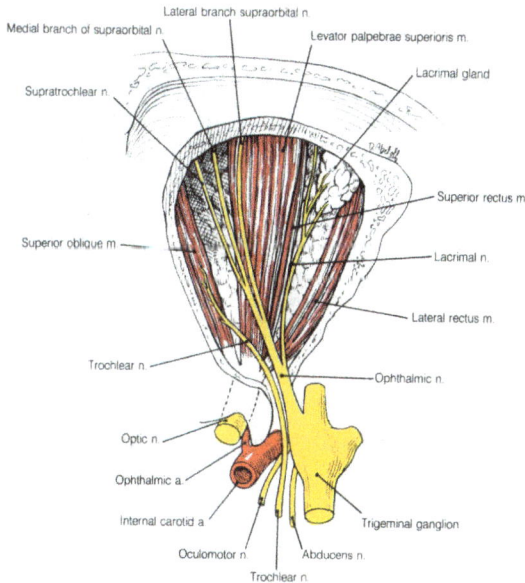

Lateral branch supraorbital n.
Medial branch of supraorbital n.
Levator palpebrae superioris m.
Lacrimal gland
Supratrochlear n.
Superior rectus m.
Superior oblique m.
Lacrimal n.
Lateral rectus m.
Trochlear n.
Ophthalmic n.
Optic n.
Ophthalmic a.
Internal carotid a.
Trigeminal ganglion
Oculomotor n.
Abducens n.
Trochlear n.

The sensory ganglion of the trigeminal nerve is sometimes still known as the semilunar ganglion, to reflect its shape, or as the Gasserian ganglion, to honor Johann Gasser.

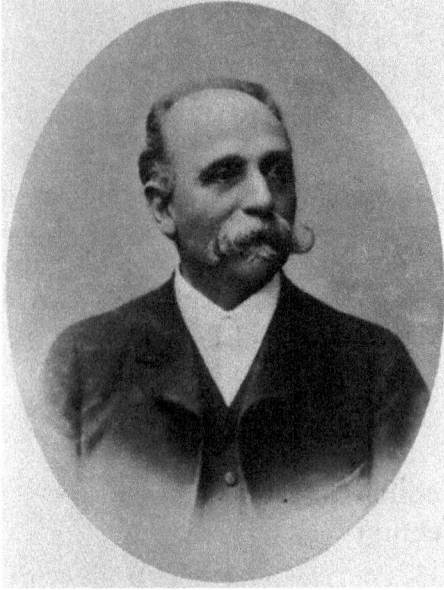

Camillo Golgi
1844-1926

Golgi, an Italian professor of histology and anatomy, shared the Nobel Prize in Physiology or Medicine in 1906 with Santiago Ramony Cajal for investigation of neurons in the central nervous system. Associated with Golgi are Golgi cells, a type of interneuron located in the cerebellum; Golgi stain, a technique of staining nerve tissue; Golgi apparatus (or complex or body), an organelle in the cell; and Golgi tendon organ, a proprioceptive sensory receptor organ.

A. J. Lantermann
19th Century

Lantermann was a member of the Strassburg Anatomical Institute in Germany. In osmium-fixed specimens of neurons and Schwann cells, the myelin sheath of the internode region is sometimes interrupted by oblique, funnel-shaped discontinuities which extend from the neurilemma to the axon. These are formed by Schwann cell cytoplasm that is not displaced to the periphery during myelin formation and are known as clefts or incisures of Schmidt-Lantermann.

Heinrich Lissauer
1861-1891

Lissauer, the son of the famous anthropologist Abraham Lissauer, was a German neurologist. The ascending tract in the spinal cord located between the entering posterior root fibers and the margin of the cord is commonly called the dorsal lateral tract of Lissauer.

Hubert Luschka
1820-1875

Luschka was a professor of anatomy in Germany. The openings at the lateral recesses of the fourth ventricle of the brain are referred to as Luschka's foramina; it is through these openings that cerebrospinal fluid flows. Luschka's joints (also known as uncovertebral joints) are located in the cervical region of the vertebral column between C3 and C6. Specifically, they are synovial joints formed between uncinate processes superiorly and the uncus inferiorly of the cervical vertebrae. These joints permit flexion and extension while limiting lateral flexion in the neck.

Francois Magendie
1783-1855

Magendie was a French professor of pathology and physiology. The median aperture of the fourth ventricle is called the Foramen of Magendie. It is through this foramen that cerebrospinal fluid flows.

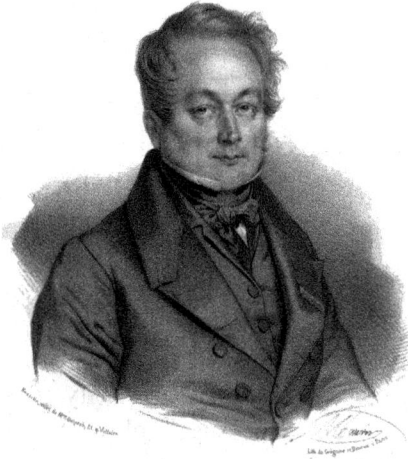

Carlo Martinotti
1859-1918

Carlo Martinotti, a student of Camillo Golgi, was recently determined to be the actual scientist who described Martinotti cells, although for years the discovery was mistakenly attributed to Giovanni Martinotti (1857-1928), an Italian pathologist and anatomist. Martinotti cells, which are scattered throughout various layers of the cerebral cortex of the brain, are small multipolar neurons with short branching dendrites.

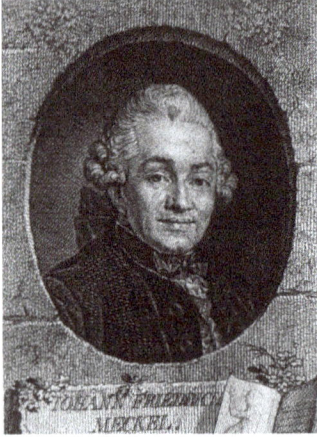

Johann Friedrich Meckel, the Elder
1724-1774

Johann Friedrich Meckel the Elder was a German professor of anatomy, botany and obstetrics. His son Philipp Friedrich Theodor Meckel, grandson August Albrecht Meckel, and grandson Johann Friedrich Meckel the Younger were also anatomists. He is credited with the discovery of the submandibular ganglion. He is associated with Meckel's cave, or space, a depression in the dura mater over the petrous portion of the temporal bone that covers the trigeminal ganglion. His name has also been associated with the pterygopalatine ganglion, which was formerly known as Meckel's ganglion, and Meckel's ligament, which attaches the malleus to the wall of the tympanic membrane.

Georg Meissner
1829-1905

Meissner was a German professor of anatomy, physiology and zoology. Meissner's corpuscles are nerve endings in the dermis and serve as mechanoreceptors, primarily sensitive to light touch. Meissner's plexus, also known as the submucosal plexus, is a collection of parasympathetic postganglionic cell bodies in the submucosa of the intestinal tract and contributes to the control of peristalsis.

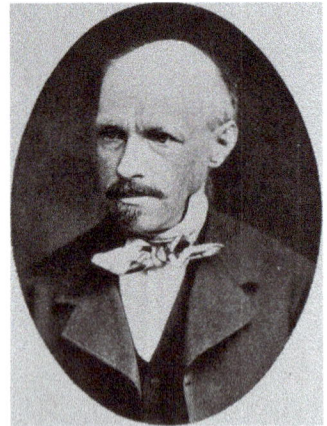

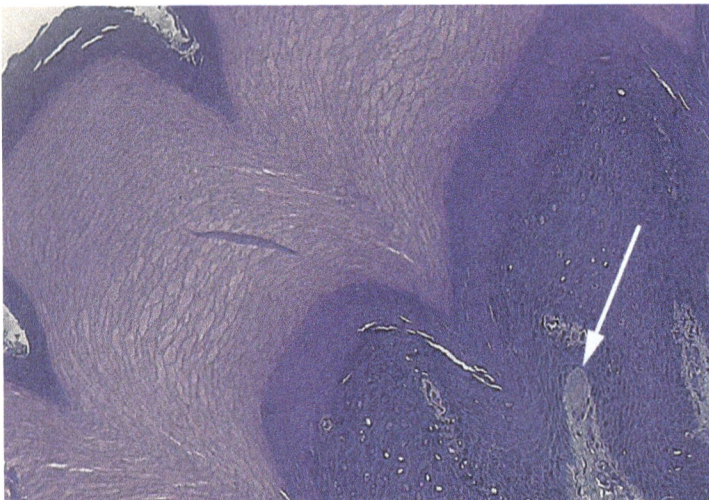

At the tip of the arrow is seen Meissner's corpuscle, nestled in a dermal papilla that interdigitates with the epidermis of the skin.

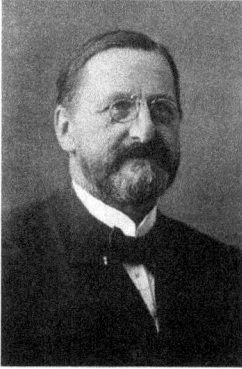

Friedrich Sigmund Merkel
1845-1919

Merkel was a German professor of anatomy. Sensory mechanoreceptors located in the stratum basale of the epidermis and receiving afferent nerve terminals are sometimes referred to as Merkel cells.

Alexander Monro (Secundus)
1733-1817

Monro (Secundus, middle) followed his father, Monro (Primus, left), as Chair of Anatomy in Edinburgh. His son, Monro (Tertius, right), was an anatomist, as well. Credit is given to Alexander Monro for the discovery of the interventricular foramen which connects the lateral ventricles with the third ventricle. We currently refer to this foramen as the foramen of Monro.

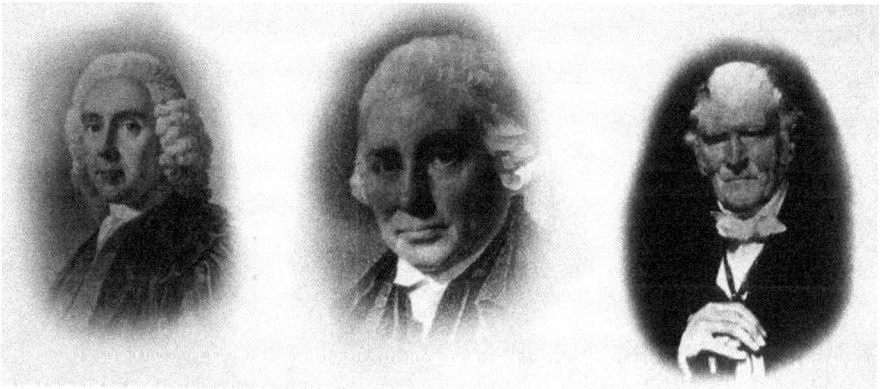

Franz Nissl
1860-1919

Nissl was a German neurologist. Clumps of basophilic material observed in the perikarya of most nerve cells are known as Nissl bodies. Nissl bodies are known to be orderly arrays of granular endoplasmic reticulum.

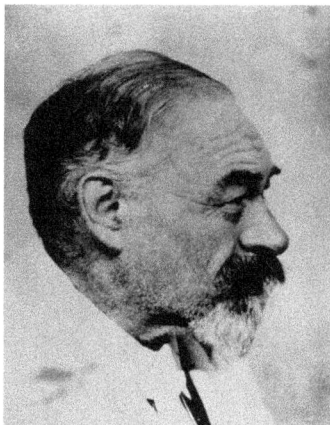

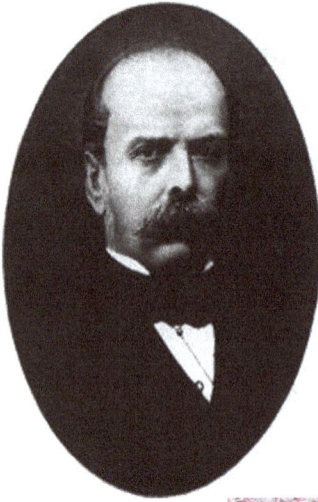

Filippo Pacini
1812-1883

Pacini was an Italian anatomist and histologist. The Pacinian corpuscle, which is located primarily in the dermis of the skin, consists of a single axon that loses its myelin sheath and is encapsulated by several layers of flattened cells with greatly attenuated cytoplasm. Its function is related to the perception of pressure, touch, and vibration.

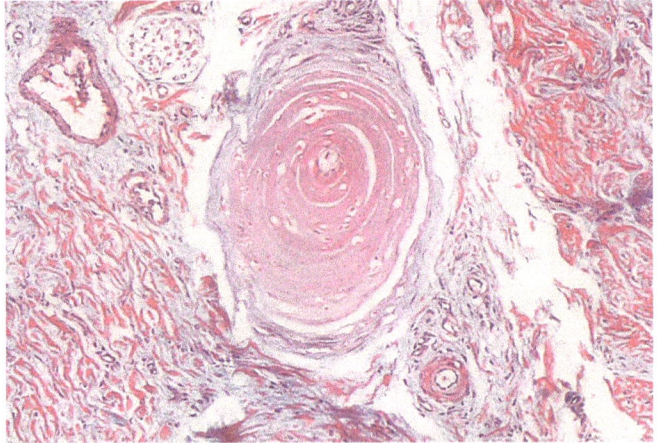

The swirled structure is a Pacinian corpuscle in the dermis of the skin.

Johannes Evangelista Purkinje
1787-1869

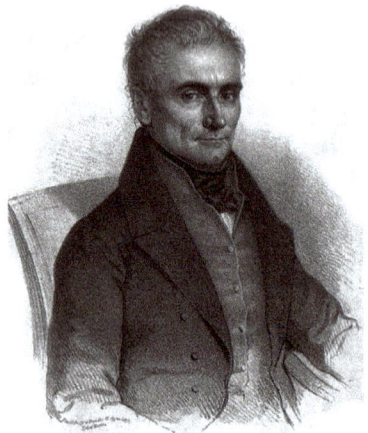

Purkinje, a physiologist and anatomist, was born in Bohemia (now in the Czech Republic) and spent his life in Breslau (now in Poland) and Prague (now in the Czech Republic). The large cells of the cerebellum with axons extending to the central cerebellar nuclei are referred to as Purkinje cells. Purkinje fibers, which are specialised myocardial cells in the heart, are located in the inner ventricular walls.

They conduct an electrical impulse, thus allowing the heart to contract in a coordinated fashion.

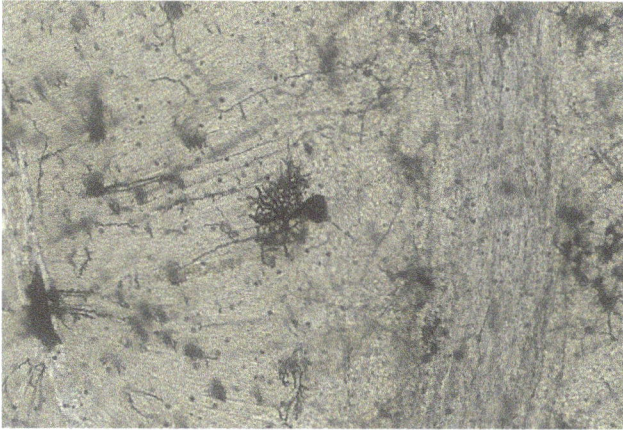

At the center of this image can be seen a cerebellar Purkinje cell, which is arborised with numerous dendrites.

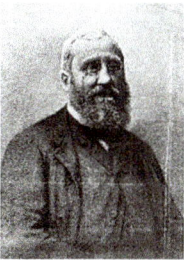

Louis Antoine Ranvier
1835-1922

Ranvier was a French physician and histologist. In nerve tissue, nodes of Ranvier are regions along the axons that lack myelin and represent discontinuities between two adjacent Schwann cells.

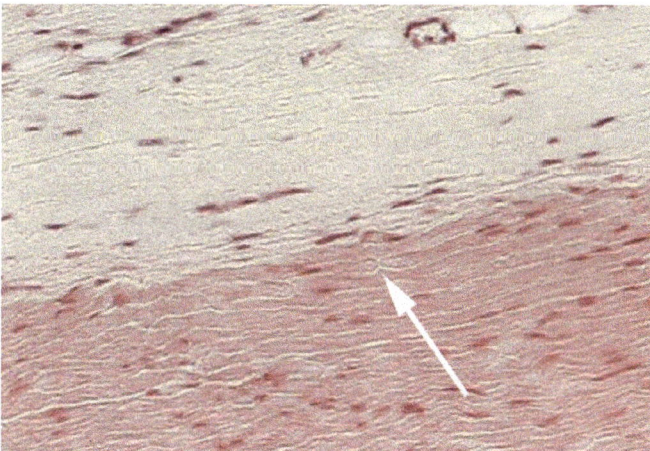

The indented region at the tip of the arrow represents the space between two adjacent Scwann cells as they surround the axon of a neuron.

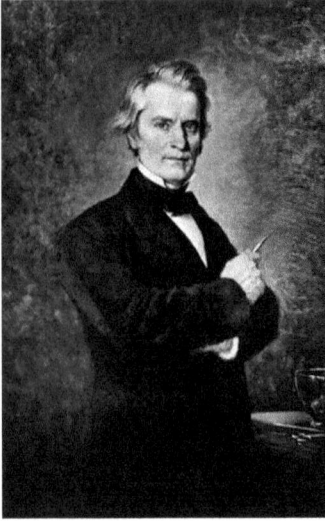

Andreas Adolf Retzius
1796-1860

Retzius was a Swedish anatomist and anthropologist. His son, Gustav Magnus Retzius, was an anatomist and neurologist. The gyri of Retzius, convolutions located in the cingulated gyrus of the brain, were named by the son in honor of the father. The most superficial layer of the cerebral cortex contain cells commonly referred to as the Retzius-Cajal cells.

Luigi Rolando
1773-1831

Rolando was an Italian anatomist. The sulcus that separates the frontal and parietal lobes of the cerebral hemispheres is known as the central sulcus of Rolando. The gelatinous substance located in the dorsal gray columns of the spinal cord is called the substantia gelatinosa of Rolando.

Angelo Ruffini
1874-1929

Ruffini was an Italian histologist. In the dermis as well as in joints, Ruffini's endings are encapsulated receptors that are composed of groups of branched nerve terminals from myelinated nerve fibers surrounded by a thin capsule of connective tissue. They serve as pressure and touch receptors.

Henry D. Schmidt
1823-1888

Schmidt was an American pathologist at the Charity Hospital in New Orleans, Louisiana. In osmium-fixed specimens of neurons and Schwann cells, the myelin sheath of the internode region is sometimes interrupted by oblique, funnel-shaped discontinuities which extend from the neurilemma to the axon. These are formed by Schwann cell cytoplasm that is not displaced to the periphery during myelin formation and are known as clefts or incisures of Schmidt-Lantermann.

Theodor Schwann
1810-1882

Schwann was a German anatomy professor who was an early supporter of the cellular doctrine of tissues. He is well known for his work with neurons. The cell responsible for the formation of myelin in the peripheral nervous system is the Schwann cell. Schwann cells can be observed wrapping around the axons of nerves.

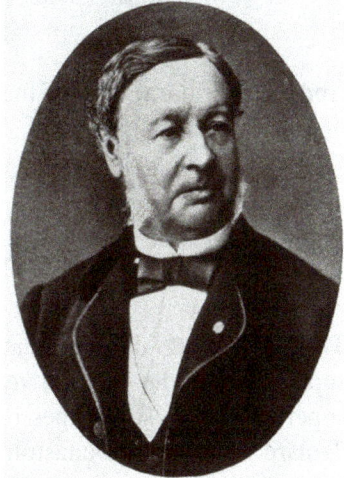

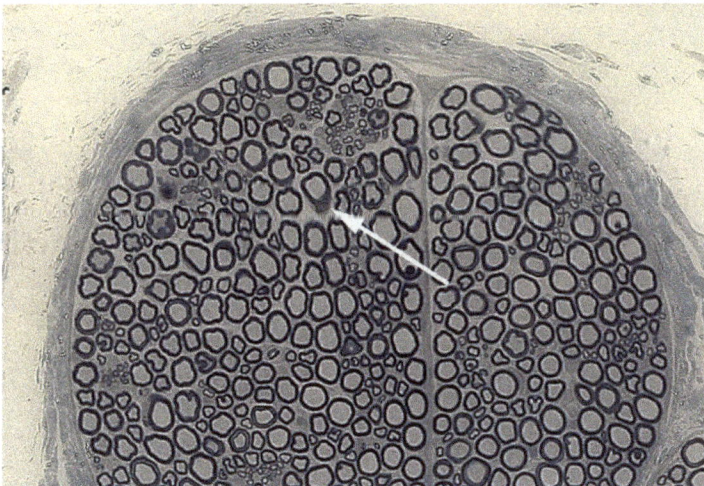

The cross section of a nerve is seen with the numerous smaller circles within it representing the myelinated axons of nerve cells that are traveling out of the plane of the page. The dark spot at the arrow is the nucleus of a Schwann cell myelinating an individual axon.

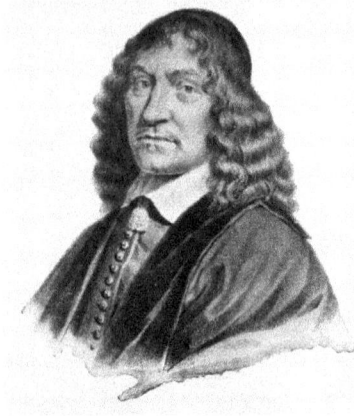

Franciscus Sylvius
1614-1672

Sylvius, born Franz de la Boe, was a Dutch physician and anatomist. He is not to be confused with Jacques Sylvius, a 15th-century French anatomist who was a teacher of Vesalius. The aperture that joins the third and fourth ventricles of the brain is commonly referred to as the cerebral aqueduct of Sylvius. The fissure separating the frontal and parietal lobes from the temporal lobe of the brain is known as the lateral cerebral fissure or fissure of Sylvius.

Paulin Trolard
1842-1910

Trolard was an Algerian anatomist. The superior anastomotic vein of the superficial middle cerebral vein drains into the superior sagittal sinus. This superior vein is sometimes referred to as the "great annectant" or vein of Trolard. The inferior anastomotic vein of Labbe empties into the transverse sinus.

Constantius Varolius
1543-1575

Varolius was an Italian anatomy professor who served as physician to Pope Gregory XIII. He studied the pons of the brain in detail, and some of the older textbooks of neuroanatomy refer to it as the pons of Varolius.

Guido Vidius
1508-1569

Vidus Vidius, born Guido Guidi, was an Italian surgeon, anatomist and author of one of the best illustrated surgical books of the 16th century. The nerve of the pterygoid canal, commonly known as the vidian nerve, is formed by the greater petrosal nerve and the deep petrosal nerve. It innervates lacrimal, nasal and palatine glands, as well as the palate with respect to taste and sensation.

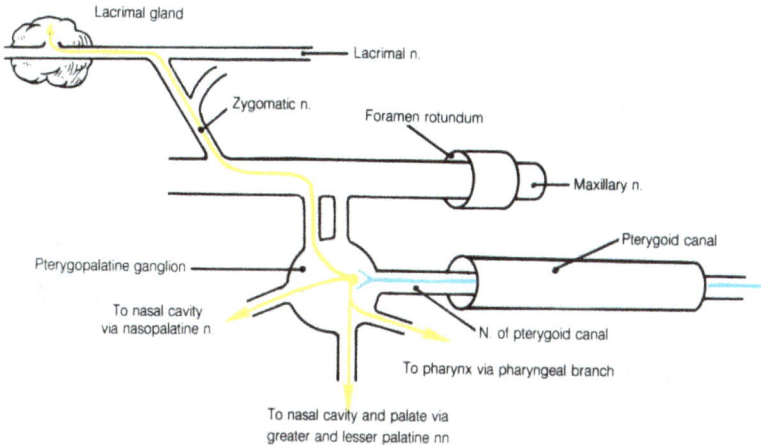

The nerve of the pterygoid canal is sometimes still called the vidian nerve.

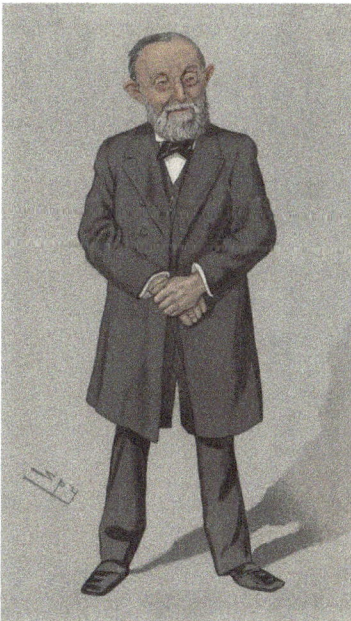

Rudolf Ludwig Karl Virchow
1821-1902

Virchow, a student of Johannes Muller, was a German anatomist and pathologist (and politician) who founded the journal *Archiv.* He is often known as the "father of modern pathology" and as a founder of social medicine. In addition to understanding that mitosis was important for cell formation ("Virchow's cell theory"), his name is used frequently throughout medical nomenclature. Of the many structures or procedures named for him, the most prominent may be the perivascular spaces that surround the blood vessels as they enter the brain substance, known as Virchow-Robin spaces.

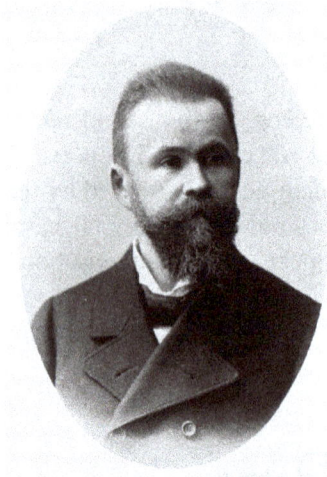

Karl Wernicke
1848-1905

Wernicke was a German neurologist and psychiatrist. Wernicke discovered that damage to the left posterior, superior temporal gyrus of the brain resulted in deficits in language comprehension, and so this region is now referred to as Wernicke's area.

Karl Friedrich Otto Westphal
1833-1890

Westphal, a German, was a neurologist and psychiatrist who was Director of the Brain Institute in Berlin. The preganglionic parasympathetic cell bodies of the oculomotor nerve, located in the mesencephalon, are referred to as the Edinger-Westphal nucleus.

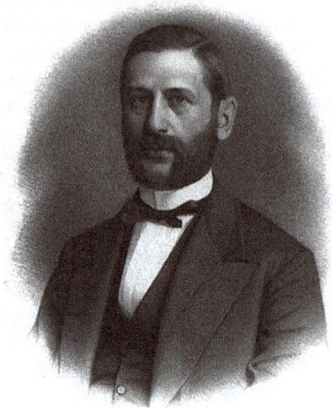

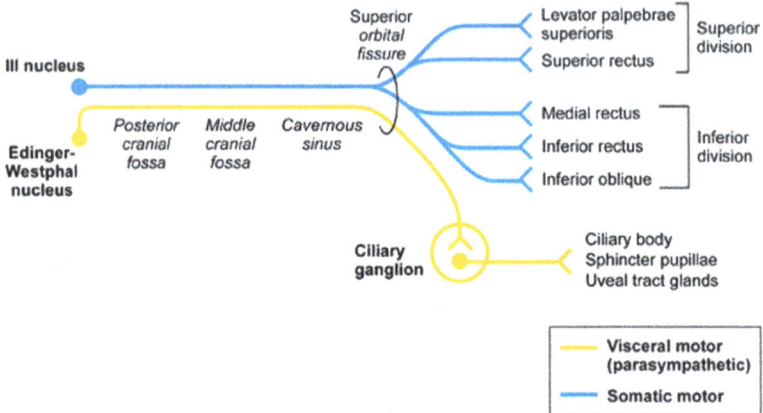

The Edinger-Westphal nucleus in the brainstem is the origin of parasympathetic neurons of the oculomotor nerve.

Thomas Willis
1621-1675

Willis, whose date of birth is sometimes given as 1622, was an English physician who cofounded the Royal Society and served as physician to James II. The arterial circle located at the base of the brain is frequently called the Circle of Willis.

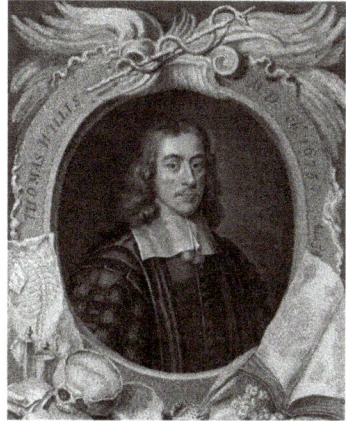

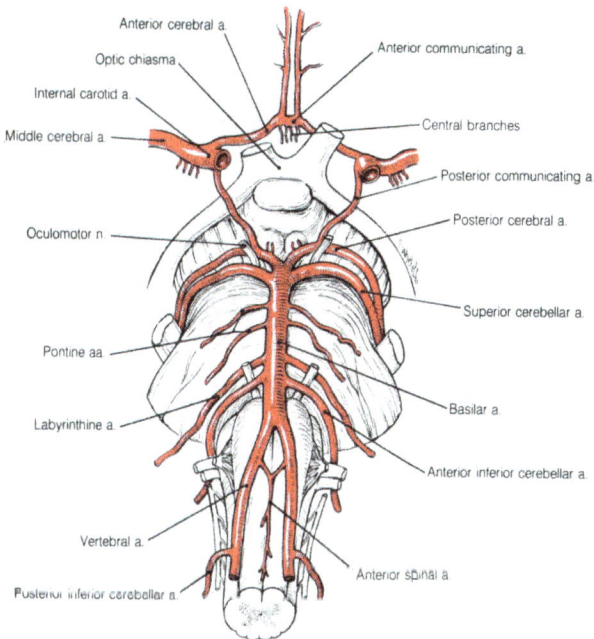

The cerebral arterial circle, or Circle of Willis, is composed of the anterior and posterior cerebral arteries as well as the anterior and posterior communicating arteries.

ENDOCRINE SYSTEM

Arthur Hill Hassall
1817-1894

Hassall was an English physician. Hassall's corpuscles are found in the medulla of the thymus and are formed from dead epithelial reticular cells arranged concentrically. The function of these structures is currently unclear.

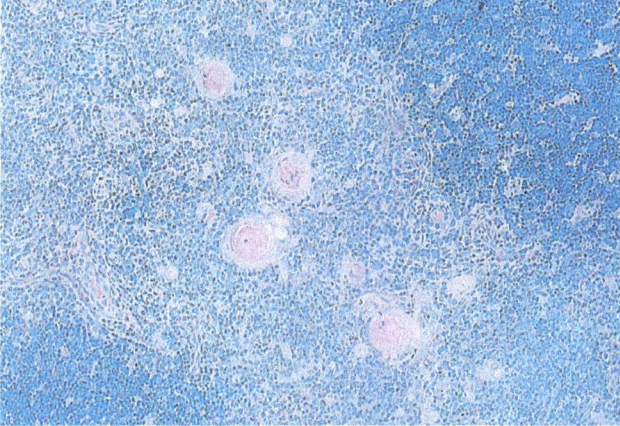

The light blue swirled regions are Hassall's corpuscles in the thymus.

Percy Theodore Herring
1872-1967

Herring was an English physician and physiologist who was a professor in Scotland. The posterior part of the pituitary gland contains tightly packed, large, unmyelinated neurons, the axons and terminals of which contain neurosecretory granules. Larger clusters of these granules are known as Herring bodies and contain either oxytocin or vasopressin.

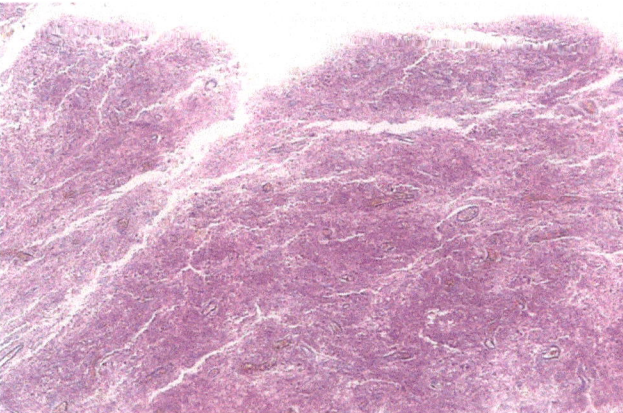

Herring bodies are clusters of granules in the posterior pituitary gland. They are seen in this image as small dark specks.

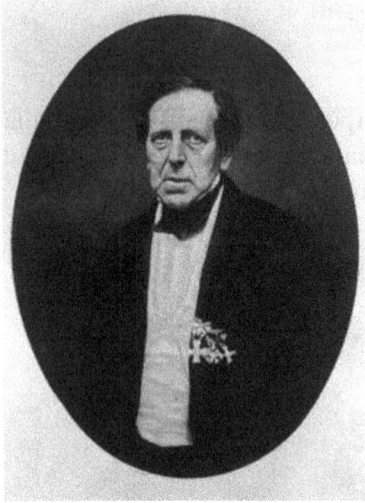

Martin Heinrich Rathke
1793-1860

Rathke was a Prussian physiologist and pathologist who lived in areas that are now included in Poland, Estonia, and Russia. A depression in the roof of the embryonic oral cavity located anterior to the buccopharyngeal membrane is known as Rathke's Pouch, which gives rise to the anterior part of the pituitary gland during development.

CARDIOVASCULAR SYSTEM

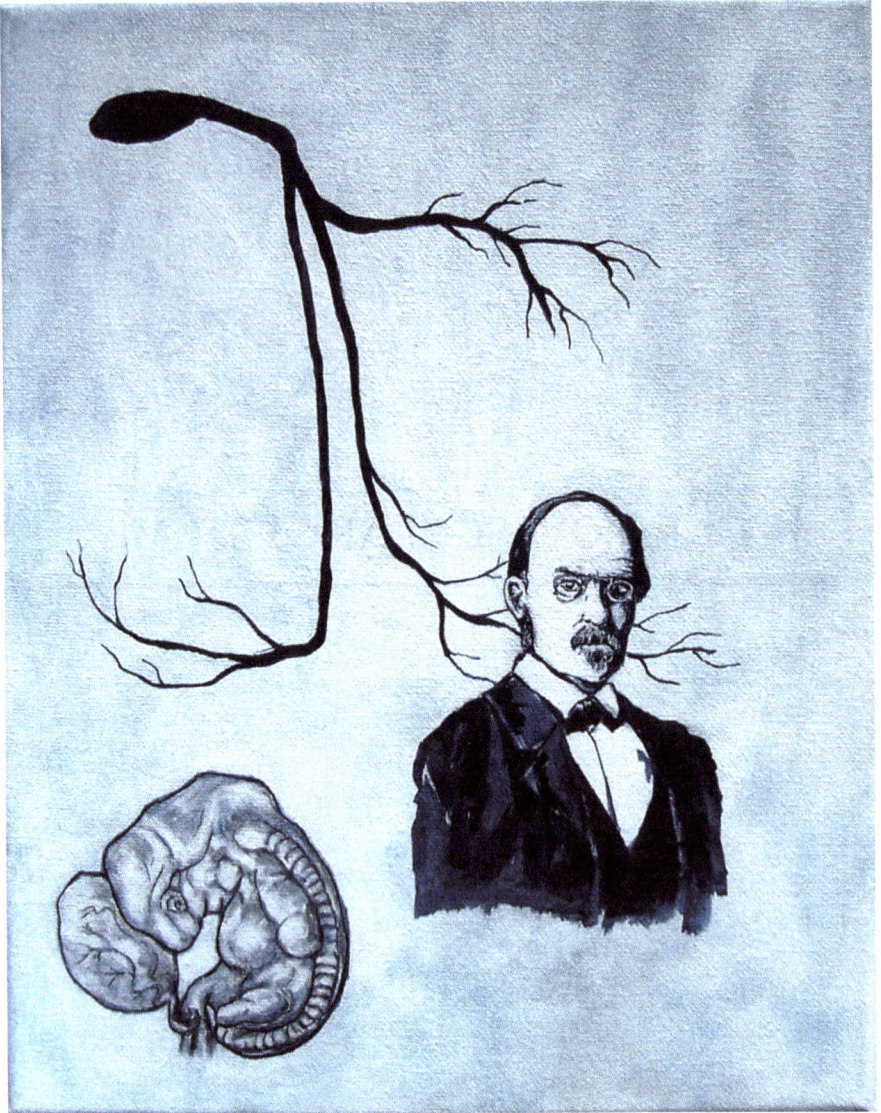

Wilhelm His, Junior
Taken from The Alphabet of Anatomical Eponyms ©Meredith Browne
http://meredithbrowne.weebly.com/alphabet-of-anatomical-eponyms.html

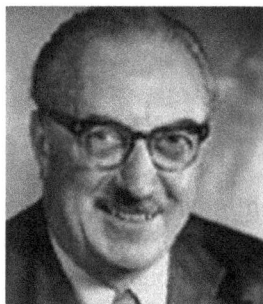

Murray Barr
1908-1995

Barr was a Canadian physician and biomedical scientist. He discovered the Barr body, which is the inactive X chromosome that can be seen on the nucleus of neutrophils.

Wilhelm His, Junior
1863-1934

His, Jr. was a German professor of anatomy. His father, Wilhelm His, Sr., studied cells that form blood vessels. The atrioventricular bundle of His is a band of conducting tissue radiating from the atrioventricular node into the interventricular septum where it divides into two branches, enters the subendocardium and continues as Purkinje fibers.

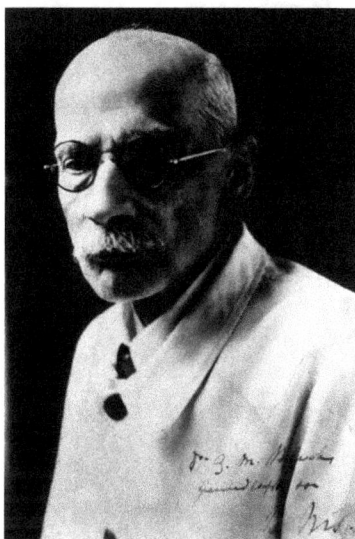

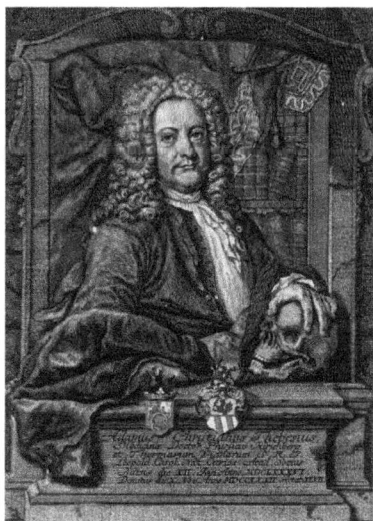

Adam Christian Thebesius
1686-1732

Thebesius was an anatomist and pathologist in what is now the Netherlands. The Thebesian valve is a one-cusp semicircular fold of tissue that marks the opening of the coronary sinus in the right atrium.

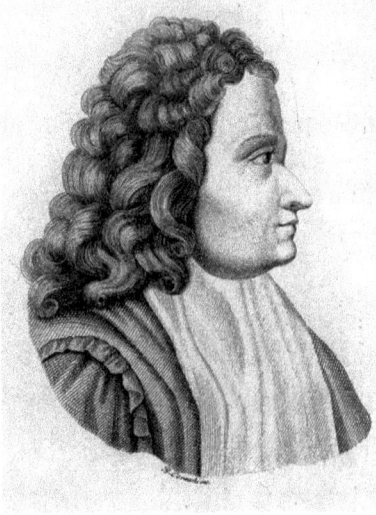

Antonia Valsalva
1666-1723

Valsalva, whose birth date is sometimes recorded as 1660, was an Italian who succeeded Marcello Malpighi as chair of anatomy at Bologna. Valsalva in turn trained Giovanni Battista Morgagni. The aortic sinuses are referred to as Valsalva's sinuses.

RESPIRATORY SYSTEM

Adam

In the book of Genesis in the Bible, Adam ate the apple, the forbidden fruit given to him by Eve in the Garden of Eden. Thus the laryngeal prominence as seen in the anterior aspect of the neck is known as the Adam's apple.

Max Clara
20th Century

Max Clara, an anatomist who was both a German and a Nazi, described Clara cells in 1937. He quite controversially used tissue from executed victims of the Third Reich for his research. Clara cells, which are located in terminal bronchioles of the lung, are noncilated cells which secrete glycosaminoglycans to protect the bronchiolar lining. They also metabolise airborne toxins.

Wilhelm Kiesselbach
1839-1902

Kiesselbach was a German otologist, rhinologist and laryngologist. The mucosa of the nasal septum presents an area that is commonly involved in nasal hemorrhage and is referred to as Kiesselbach's area.

Hans Kohn
1866-1935

Kohn was a German physician. Alveolar pores of Kohn are openings between adjacent alveoli of the lungs and function as a means of collateral ventilation.

Francis Sibson
1814-1876

Sibson was Professor of Medicine at St. Mary's Hospital in London, England. The cervical pleura of the lung projects into the neck above the first rib and is reinforced by Sibson's fascia, which is a thickened portion of the endothoracic fascia.

DIGESTIVE SYSTEM

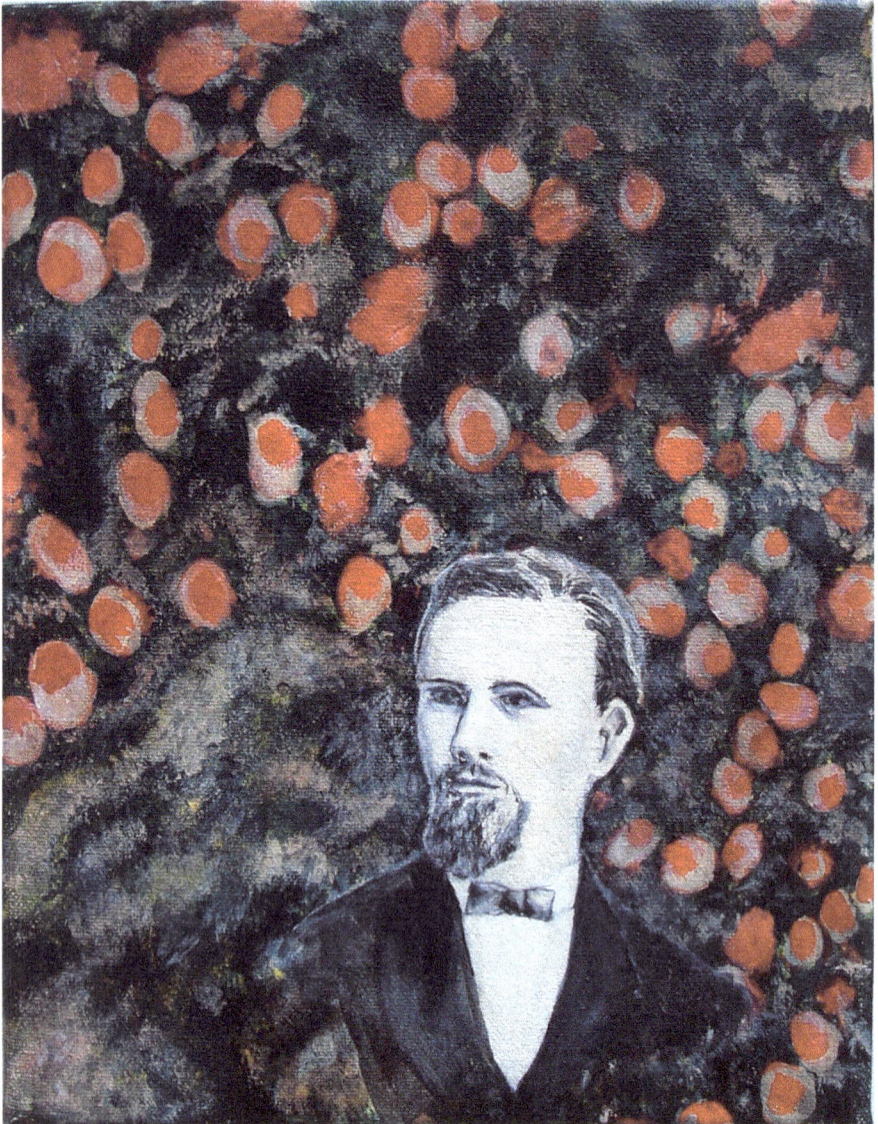

Paul Langerhans
Taken from The Alphabet of Anatomical Eponyms ©Meredith Browne
http://meredithbrowne.weebly.com/alphabet-of-anatomical-eponyms.html

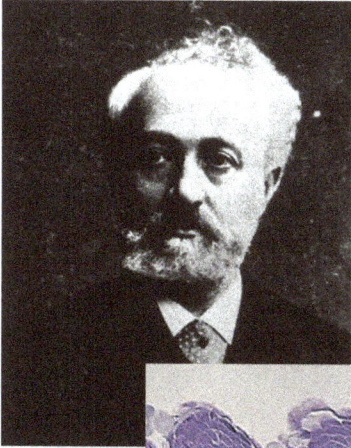

Leopold Auerbach
1828-1897

Auerbach, who was born in Poland, was a professor of neuropathology in Germany. The parasympathetic nerves that supply the stomach and intestines form a plexus that is located between the layers of smooth muscle. It is known as the myenteric plexus or Auerbach's plexus.

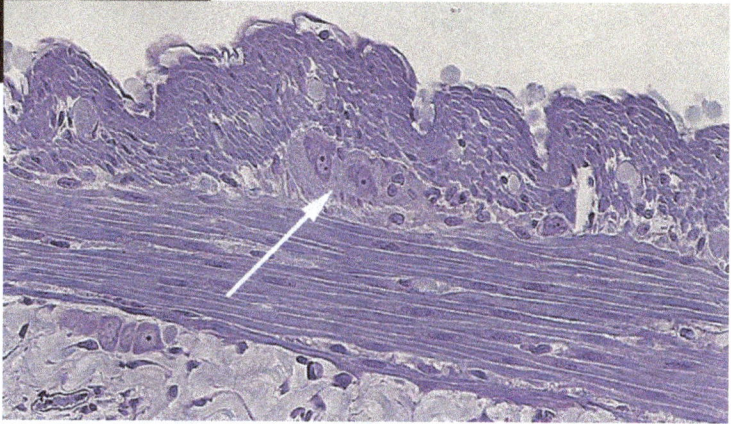

The parasympathetic neurons at the arrow are known as the myenteric plexus or Auerbach's plexus. They lie between two layers of smooth muscle in the gut. The space at the top of the image represents the peritoneal cavity.

Christian Albert Theodore Billroth
1829-1894

Billroth, born in Prussia, was a surgeon and anatomist in Switzerland and Austria. The red pulp of the spleen is traversed by a plexus of venous sinuses by which it is broken into anastomosing cords called pulp cords of Billroth. Although the spleen is an organ of the lymphoid system and not the digestive system, it is often considered with these organs because of its embryological origin.

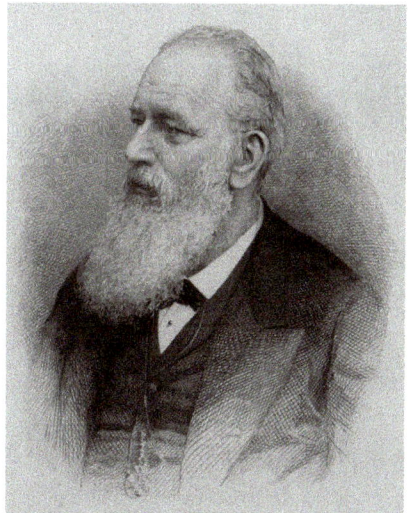

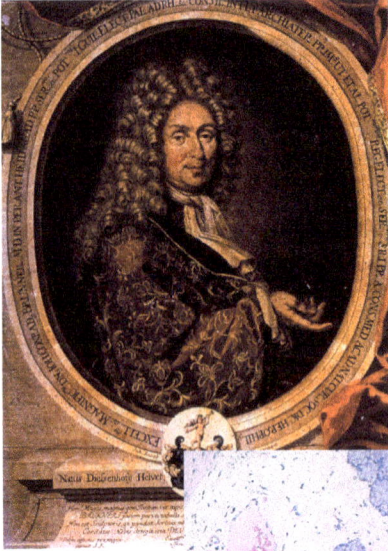

Johann Konrad Brunner
1653-1727

Brunner was born in Switzerland and educated in Paris. He later became Professor of Anatomy in Germany. The most distinguishing characteristic of the upper duodenum are the duodenal glands of Brunner in the submucosa. These glands produce an alkaline fluid to neutralise hydrochloric acid from the stomach.

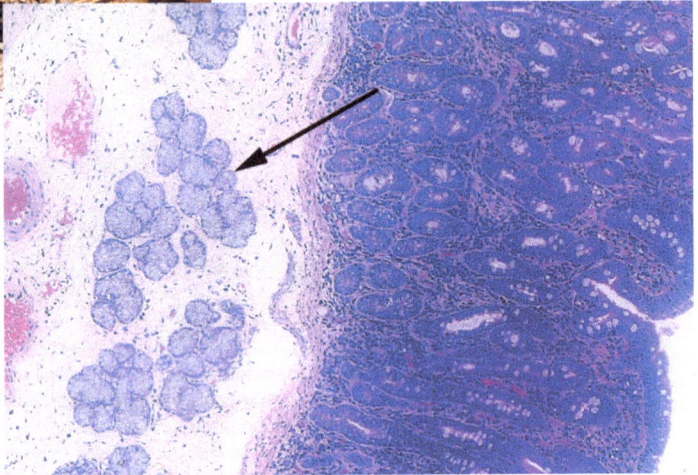

The light blue clusters at the arrow are Brunner's glands of the duodenum of the small intestine. The lumen of the duodenum is barely seen at the right.

Joseph Disse
1852-1912

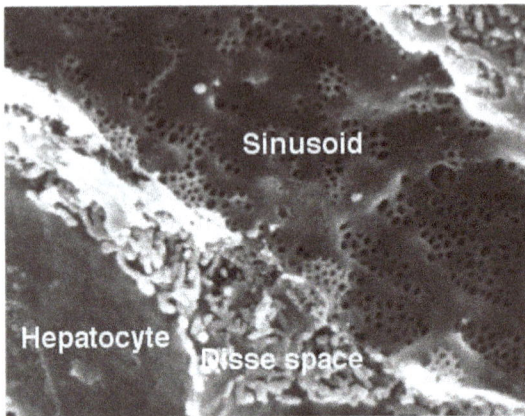

The space of Disse is located between the hepatocytes and the sinusoids, or large capillaries, in the liver.

Disse was a German histologist and anatomist. In the liver, the Space of Disse is a subendothelial (or perisinusoidal) space located between hepatocytes and liver sinusoids. Its function is to allow the exchange of material between hepatocytes and the bloodstream.

Giuseppe Giannuzzi
19th Century

Giannuzzi was an Italian anatomist. In sublingual and submandibular salivary glands, the demilunes of Giannuzzi are crescent-shaped collections of serous cells which form a cap around mucous acini and secrete lysozyme, an antimicrobial agent.

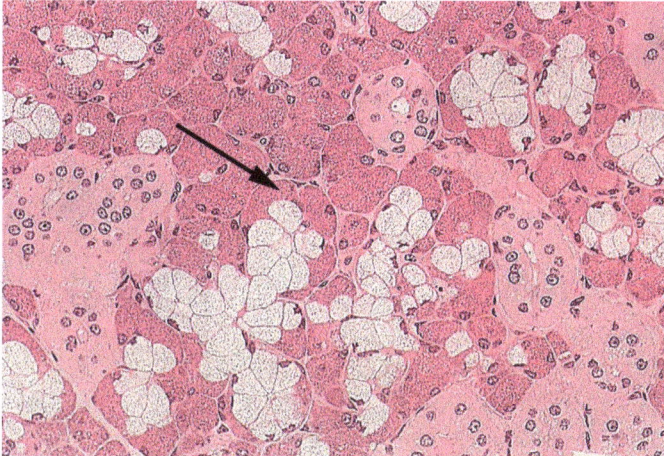

At the tip of the arrow are seen a few red cells which form a half-moon-shaped cap on top of a few pale cells. These red cells are known as serous demilunes of Giannuzzi.

Francis Glisson
1597-1677

Glisson was a physician and anatomist who was a professor in Cambridge, England. He was a founder of the Royal Society and president of the Royal College of Physicians and was also a prominent figure in the research of rickets. The fibrous capsule of the liver is commonly referred to as Glisson's capsule.

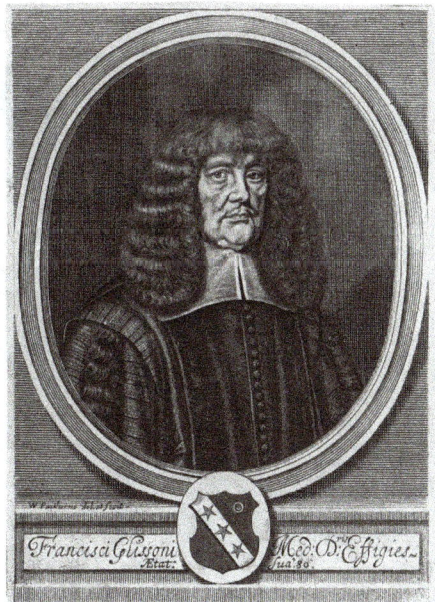

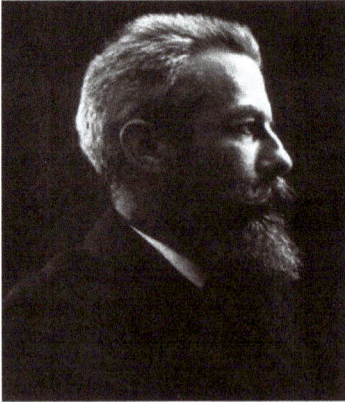

Henri Albert Charles Antoine Hartmann
1860-1936

Hartmann served as Professor of Surgery in the Faculty of Medicine in Paris, France. The location on the large intestine where the lowest branches of the sigmoid artery join with the upper branches of the superior rectal artery is referred to as Hartmann's critical point. A dilation of the neck of the gall bladder is sometimes referred to as Hartmann's pouch.

Lorenz Heister
1683-1758

Heister was an anatomist, botanist and surgeon in what is now the Netherlands. The folds in the cystic duct are often arranged in a spiral manner known as the spiral valve of Heister.

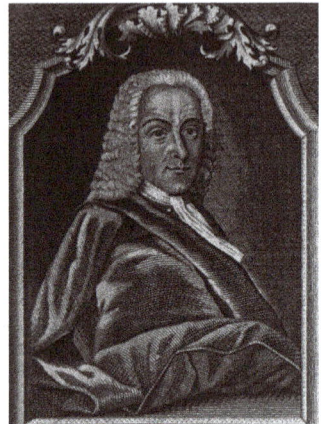

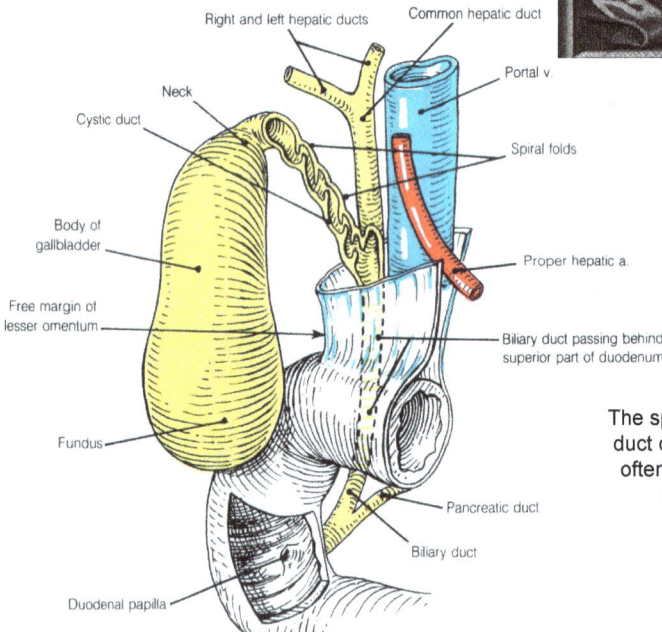

The spiral folds of the cystic duct of the gall bladder are often still called the spiral valve of Heister.

Karl Ewald Konstantin Hering
1834-1918

Ewland Hering was a German physiologist who studied color vision as well as the liver. The terminal ductules of the bile duct are sometimes referred to as the canals of Hering.

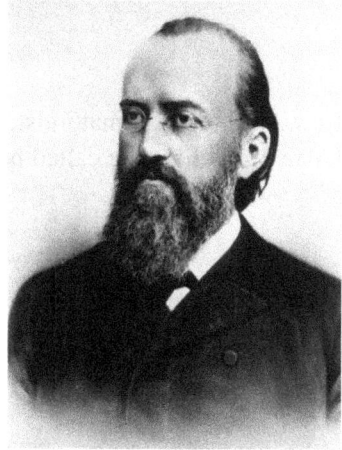

John Hilton
1805-1878

Hilton was a surgeon at Guy's Hospital in London, England. He was a Fellow of the Royal Society, a Hunterian Professor of Anatomy and an original fellow and president of the Royal College of Surgeons. The terminal end of the transitional zone of the rectum ends at a narrow wavy region, commonly called the white line of Hilton.

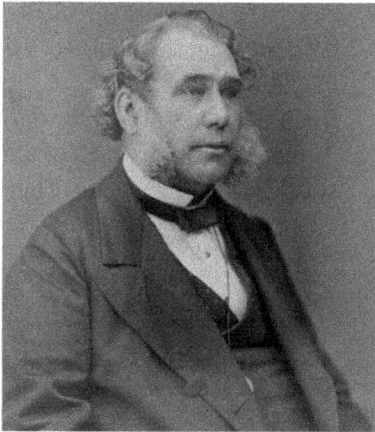

John Houston
1802-1845

Houston was a physician in Dublin, Ireland. Three transverse rectal folds are usually present; the middle fold is the more prominent and is commonly referred to as Houston's fold.

The middle of the three transverse folds of the rectum is more prominent and is known as Houston's fold.

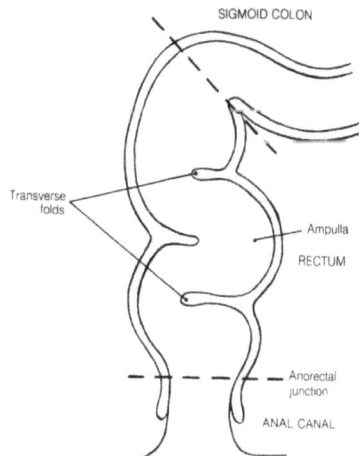

SIGMOID COLON

Transverse folds

Ampulla

RECTUM

Anorectal junction

ANAL CANAL

Toshio Ito
1904-1991

Ito was a Japanese anatomist. Fat-storing stellate cells located in the space of Disse of the liver are called hepatic lipocytes, or Ito cells.

Theodor Kerckring
1640-1693

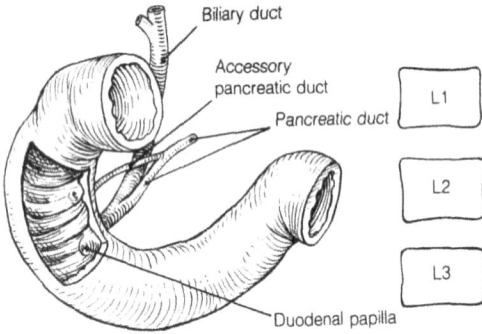

The ridges of the inner lining of the small intestine are plicae circulares – or the valves of Kerckring. They are not actually valves, however.

Kerckring was a German anatomist and physician in Amsterdam. The valves of Kerckring, or plicae circulares, are permanent spiral folds of the mucosa and submucosa of the small intestine. They serve to increase the surface area of the small intestine by a factor of ten.

Karl Wilhelm von Kupffer
1829-1902

Kupffer was a German anatomist and embryologist. Kupffer cells, located in the endothelial lining of the liver, are phagocytic cells that remove debris such as cellular fragments from the blood.

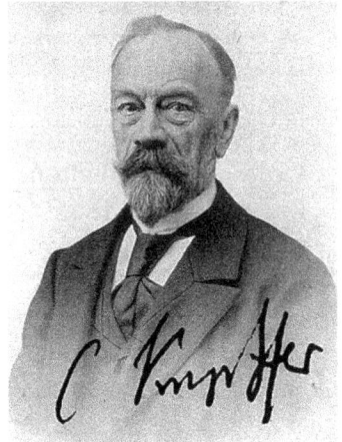

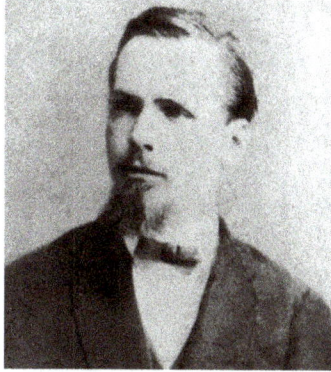

Paul Langerhans
1847-1888

Langerhans was a German physician, anatomist and pathologist. Scattered throughout the exocrine portion of the pancreas are richly-vascularised small masses of endocrine cells commonly referred to as islets of Langerhans. In the epidermis of the skin, Langerhans cells are dendritic cells which contain Birbeck granules and which function as antigen-presenting cells in immune responses.

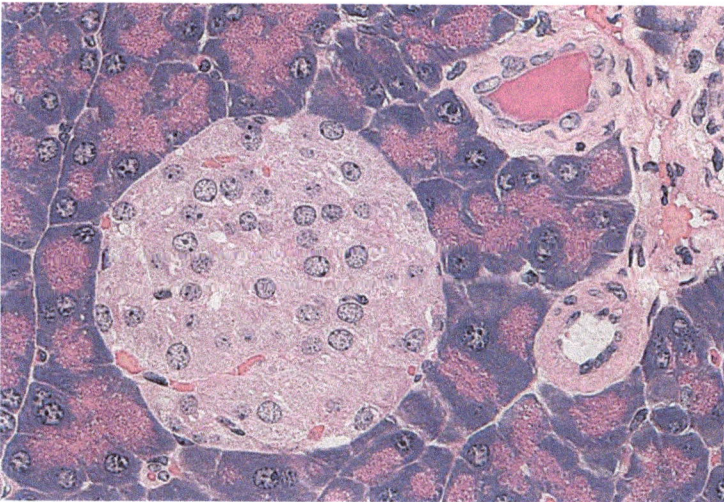

The large circular bundle of cells, known as an islet of Langerhans, produces insulin, glucagon and other hormones. Islets of Langerhans are scattered throughout the pancreas.

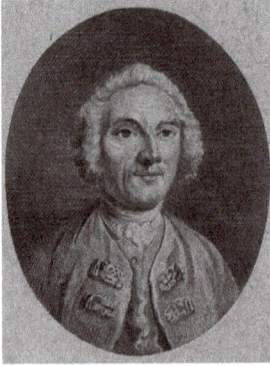

Johann Nathanael Lieberkuhn
1711-1756

Lieberkuhn was a German physician and anatomist. The crypts of Lieberkuhn are simple tubular glands, or invaginations, in the epithelium of the intestine. They are composed of goblet cells, columnar cells, enteroendocrine cells, cells that have regenerative capacity and Paneth cells.

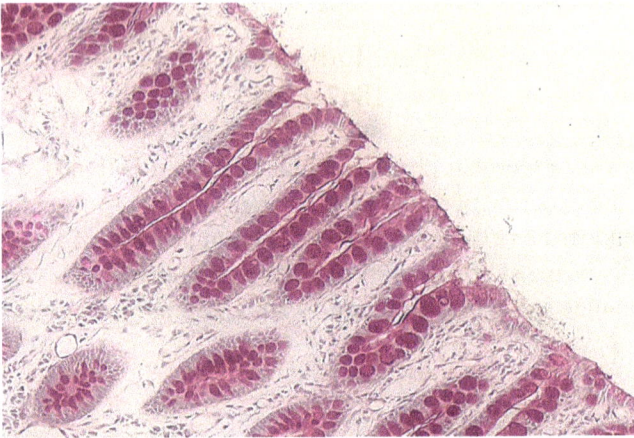

The invaginating pits are known as crypts of Lieberkuhn and are seen here in the large intestine. The large space at the upper right is the lumen of the large intestine.

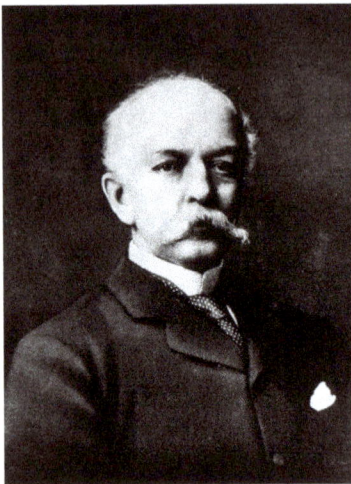

Charles McBurney
1845-1913

McBurney was a Professor of Surgery at the College of Physicians and Surgeons in New York. The base of the appendix lies deep to a point that is one-third of the way along the oblique line extending from the anterior superior iliac spine to the umbilicus. The site of maximum tenderness in cases of appendicitis is referred to as McBurney's point.

Johann Friedrich Meckel, the Younger
1781-1833

Johann Friedrich Meckel the Younger was a German professor of pathology, anatomy and surgery who was interested in birth defects. His grandfather was Johann Friedrich Meckel the Elder. Meckel's diverticulum, present in only 2% of the population, is located on the ileum and represents the remains of the vitelline duct of early fetal life. Meckel's cartilage is a cartilaginous bar from which the mandible is formed in the first pharyngeal arch of the embryo.

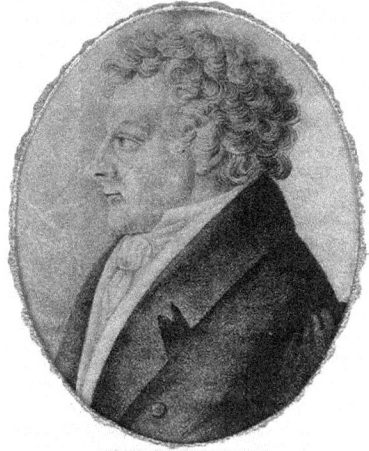

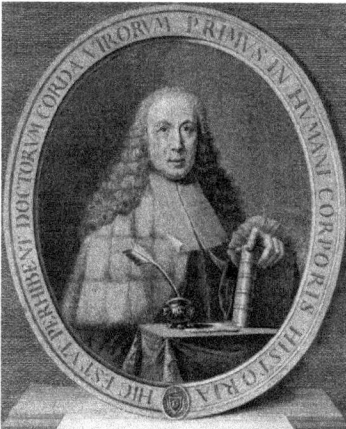

Giovanni Battista Morgagni
1682-1771

Morgagni, who studied under Antonia Maria Valsalva, was a Professor of Anatomy in Padua, Italy. He is often known as the "Father of Morbid Anatomy" (pathology). The five to ten vertical folds of anal mucous membrane are commonly referred to as anal columns of Morgagni.

James Rutherford Morison
1853-1939

Morison, an English surgeon, studied under both Lister and Billroth and specialised in abdominal surgery. The right hepatorenal recess, or space, between the inferior surface of the liver and the right kidney, is commonly referred to as the hepatorenal pouch of Morison.

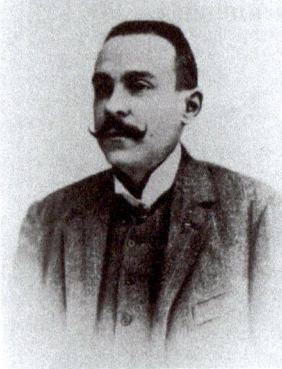

Ruggero Oddi
1864-1913

Oddi was an Italian anatomist and physiologist. The sphincter that surrounds the distal end of the common bile duct is referred to as sphincter of Oddi.

Joseph Paneth
1857-1890

Paneth was a physiologist who was on the faculty at universities in what are now Poland and Austria. Pyramidal cells with secretory granules in the apical cytoplasm, located in small groups in the depths of the crypts of Lieberkuhn, are known as Paneth cells. They secrete lysozyme, an antibacterial enzyme.

Johann Conrad Peyer
1653-1712

Peyer was a Professor of Logic, Rhetoric and Medicine in Switzerland. Peyer's patches are large continuous aggregates of lymphoid nodules in the walls of the ileum of the small intestine.

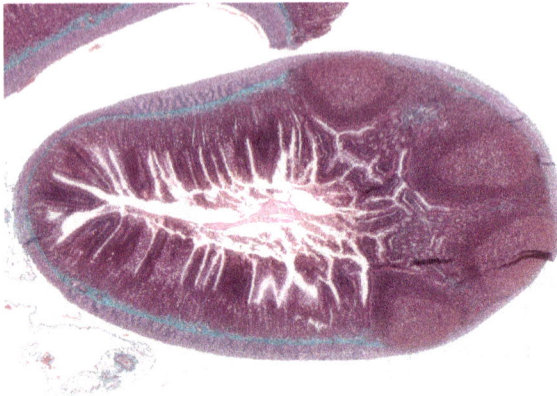

This image of a cross section of the appendix contains aggregates of lymphoid tissue on the right known as Peyer's patches.

Giandomenico Santorini
1681-1737

Santorini was an Italian professor of medicine and anatomy. The accessory duct of the pancreas is called the duct of Santorini.

Niels Stensen
1638-1686

Stensen was born in Denmark and later studied under Bartholin and Sylvius. Sometimes known as the "Father of Geology," he studied crystals as well as muscle and brain. He was a professor of anatomy in Copenhagen before becoming titular Bishop of Titiopolis, appointed by Pope Innocent XII. The parotid duct is often called Stensen's duct.

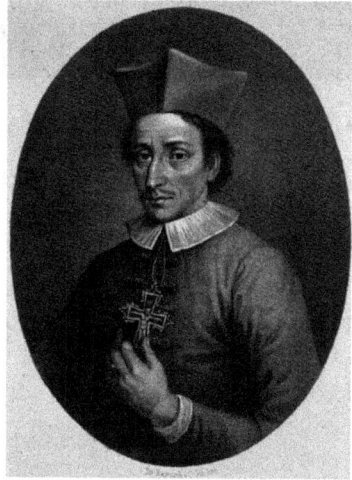

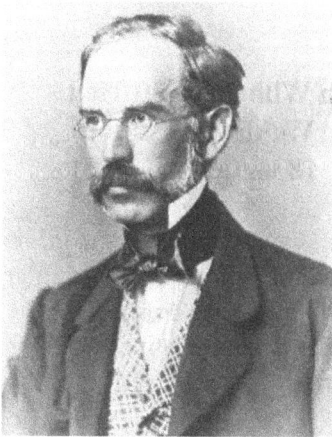

Wenzel Treitz
1819-1872

Treitz was a distinguished Austrian physician and pathologist. The small suspensory muscle of the distal end of the duodenum is commonly called the ligament of Treitz.

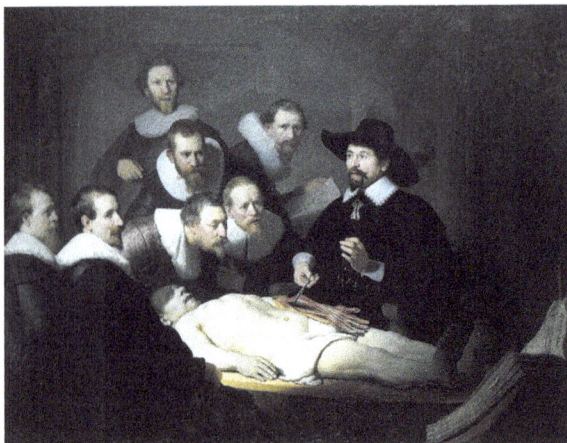

Nicolas Tulp
1593-1674

Tulp, a Dutch anatomist, is the central figure of Rembrandt's *The Lesson in Anatomy*. The ileocecal valve is referred to as Tulp's valve.

Abraham Vater
1684-1751

Vater was a professor of anatomy, botany and pathology in Wittenberg, which is now part of Germany. The ampulla of the bile duct is known as the ampulla of Vater.

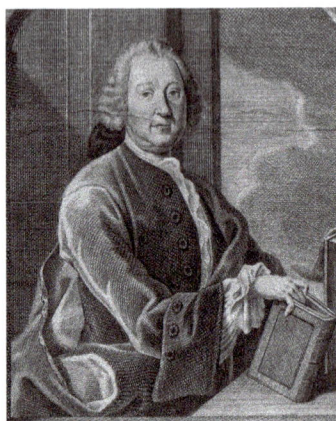

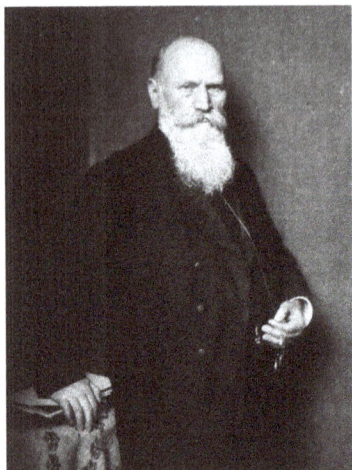

Heinrich Wilhelm Gottfried
Waldeyer
1836-1921

Waldeyer was a German anatomist, pathologist and embryologist. The circular series of lymphoid tissue formed by the lingual, pharyngeal and palatine tonsils is frequently referred to as Waldeyer's tonsillar ring.

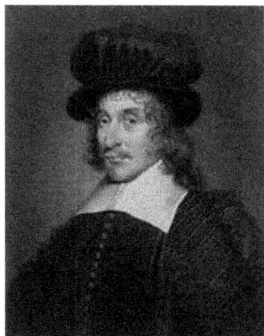

Thomas Wharton
1616-1673

Wharton, whose birth date is sometimes given as 1610 and 1614, was an English phsyician at St. Thomas's Hospital. The submandibular salivary duct is frequently referred to as Wharton's duct.

Jacob Winslow
1669-1760

Winslow, born in Denmark, was a professor of anatomy and surgery in Paris, France. The lesser peritoneal sac is a space behind the stomach which is closed off from the major peritoneal cavity (greater peritoneal sac) except for the communication through the epiploic foramen, or omental foramen, known as the foramen of Winslow.

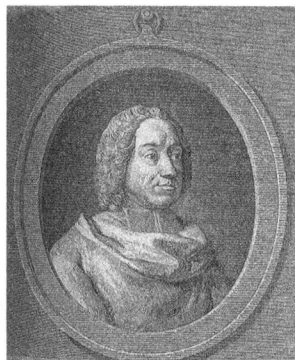

Johann Georg Wirsung
17th Century

Wirsung, born in Bavaria, was an anatomist in Italy. He was assassinated in 1643. The main pancreatic duct is commonly called the the duct of Wirsung.

URINARY SYSTEM

Lorenzo Bellini
1643-1704

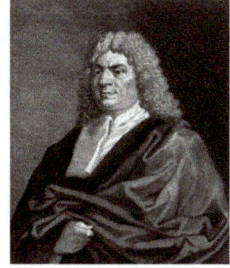

Bellini was an Italian anatomist and physician. In the inner zone of the medulla of the kidney, the papillary collecting tubules unite with other straight tubules to form the ducts of Bellini.

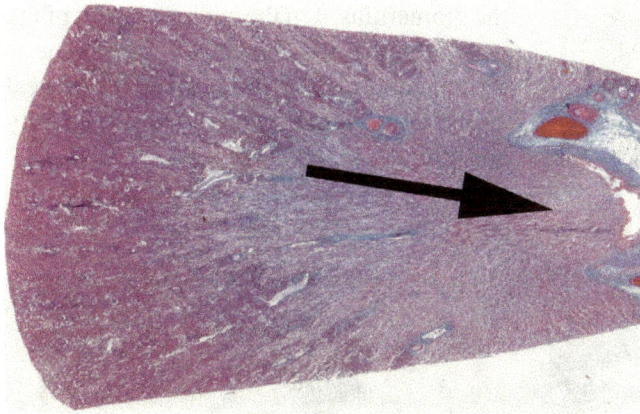

The tip of the arrow demonstrates the ducts of Bellini in the kidney. The space at the left is the area outside the kidney, and the small space at the right represents the region where urine is collected before being deposited into the ureter.

Exupere Joseph Bertin
1712-1781

Bertin was a French anatomist who studied speech, the circulatory system and the kidney. The renal columns of Bertin are extensions of cortical tissue that are located between adjacent renal pyramids.

Frontal section through the Kidney

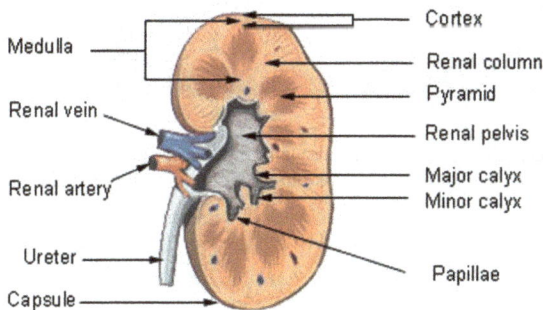

Medulla —
Renal vein —
Renal artery —
Ureter —
Capsule —

Cortex
Renal column
Pyramid
Renal pelvis
Major calyx
Minor calyx
Papillae

Extensions of the renal cortex (light regions) known as renal columns of Bertin extend in between the renal pyramids (dark regions).

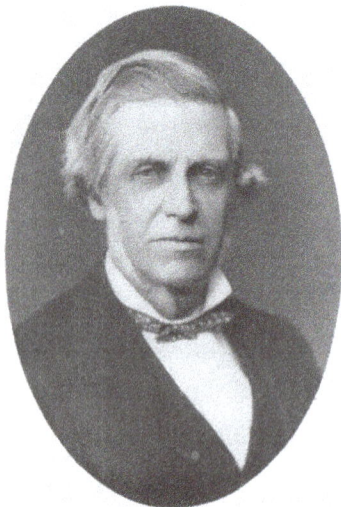

Sir William Bowman
1816-1892

Sir Bowman was an English surgeon, anatomist and physiologist who was known as the leading ophthalmic surgeon in England. In the kidney, each nephron begins in a spherical expansion, known as Bowman's capsule, which encloses a tuft of capillaries, the glomerulus. On the anterior aspect of the cornea of the eye, Bowman's membrane is the noncellular layer just beneath the corneal epithelium; its function is to provide stability and strength to the cornea.

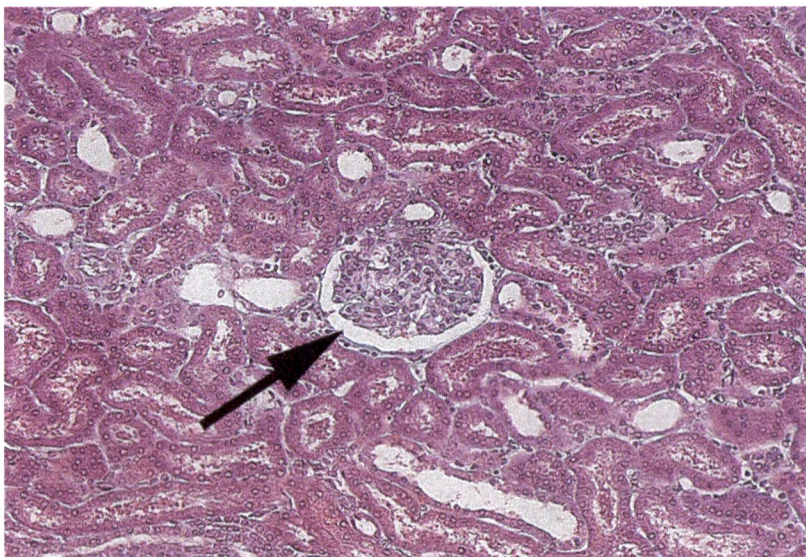

In the kidney, Bowman's capsule (arrow) is formed by a parietal and visceral layer of cells surrounding the glomerulus, the circular tuft of capillaries.

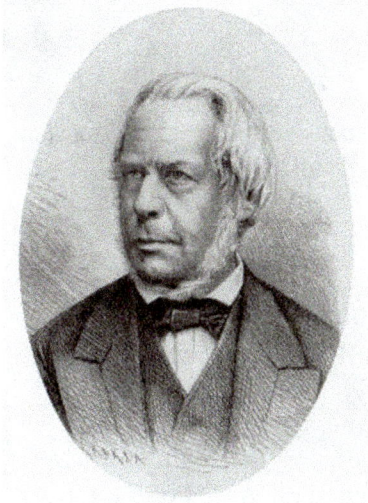

Freidrich Gustav Jakob Henle
1809-1885

Henle was a German anatomist who specialised in histology, also known as microscopic anatomy. The looped portion of a uriniferous tubule of the kidney is known as the loop of Henle. In the skin, Henle's layer, along with Huxley's layer and the cuticle, form the internal root sheath of a hair follicle.

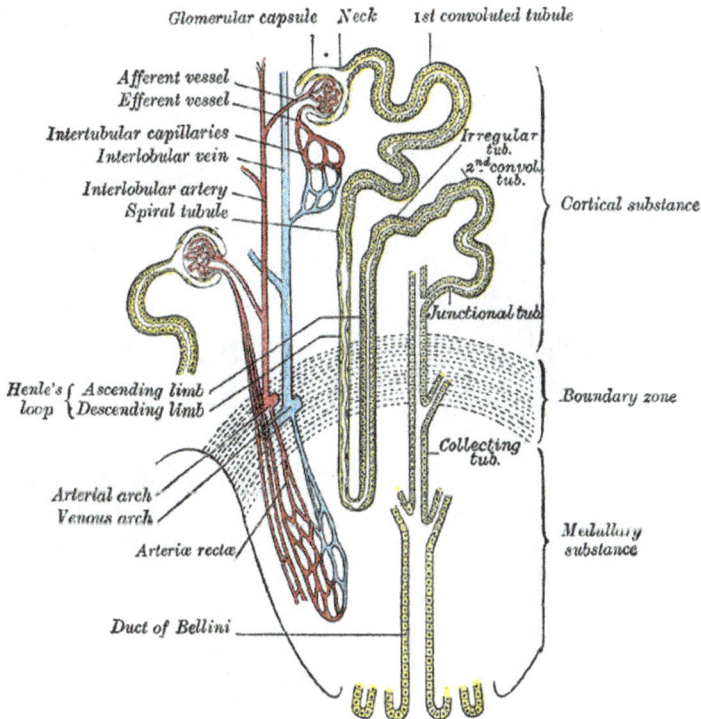

The looped portion of the uriniferous tubule of the kidney is the loop of Henle.

Alexis Littre
1658-1726

Littre was a French surgeon and anatomist. Mucus-secreting glands located in the wall of the urethra are referred to as the glands of Littre.

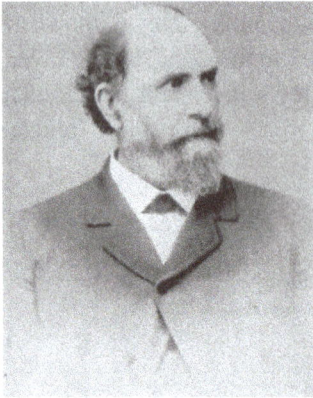

Alexander Johnston Chalmers Skene
1838-1900

Skene was a professor of gynecology in the Long Island College Hospital in Brooklyn, New York. The paraurethral glands of the female urethra are called Skene's glands.

Kaspar Friedrich Wolff
1733-1794

Wolff, a German, was a professor of anatomy and physiology in Russia. He is considered to be a

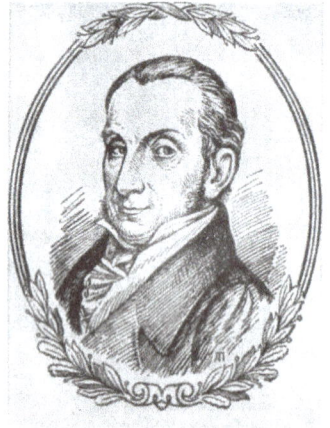

founder of modern embryology and is known for his pioneering work on the three germ layers. The development of the genital system of the male begins with the differentiation of the mesonephric or Wolffian duct.

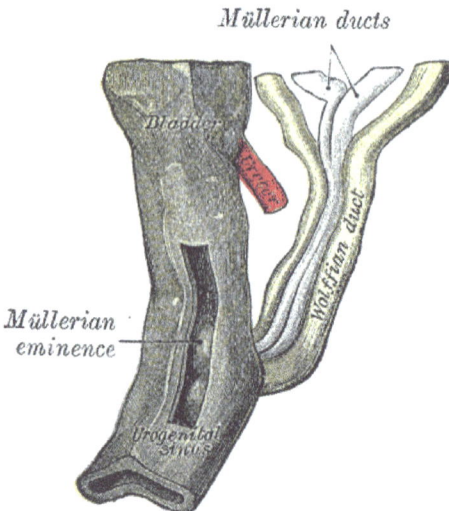

The mesonephric duct is still known as the Wolffian duct by embryologists.

REPRODUCTIVE SYSTEM

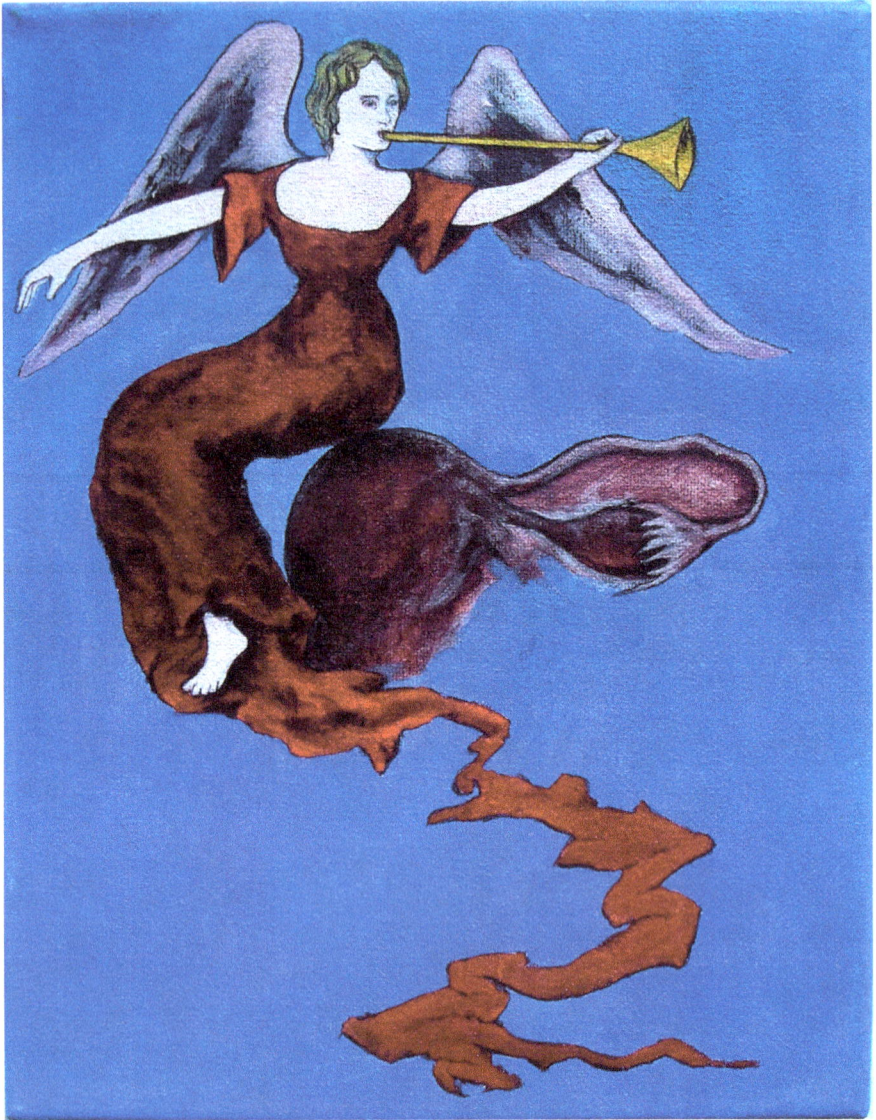

Gabriele Falloppio
Taken from *The Alphabet of Anatomical Eponyms* ©Meredith Browne
http://meredithbrowne.weebly.com/alphabet-of-anatomical-eponyms.html

Benjamin Alcock
19th Century

Alcock, an Irishman born in 1801, became a professor of anatomy, physiology and pathology. In 1853, he was asked to resign because of violations of the Anatomy Acts and traveled to the United States, where he presumably died. Alcock's canal, most often known as the pudendal canal, is located on the lateral wall of the ischiorectal fossa within the perineum. It is a fascial canal formed by a split in the fascia of the obturator internus muscle and allows the passage of the pudendal nerve and internal pudendal vessels.

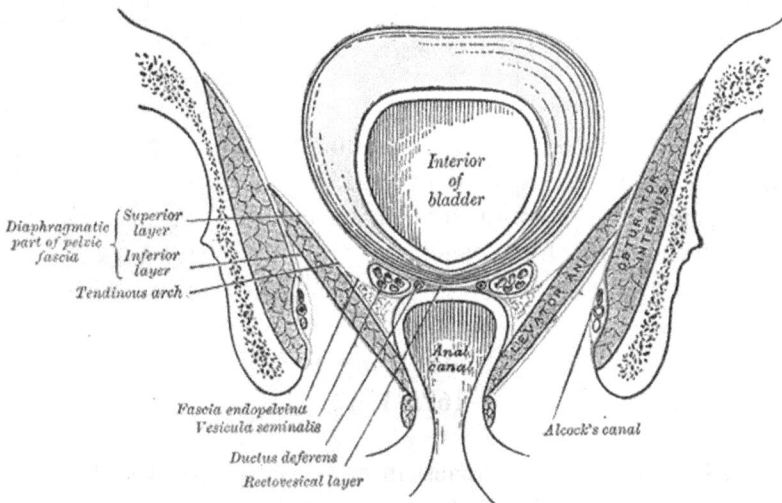

In this coronal section of the male pelvis, Alcock's canal (pudendal canal) transmits neurovasculature to the perineum.

Caspar Bartholin (Secundus)
1655-1738

Bartholin (Secundus), born in Sweden, was the son of Thomas Bartholin (Primus), who was a mathematician and anatomist who discovered the thoracic duct and lymphatic system. Bartholin was a professor of medicine, anatomy and physics in Copenhagen, Denmark. Bartholin's glands (or greater vestibular glands) are two glands located slightly below, and lateral to, the opening of the vagina. They secrete mucus to lubricate the vagina and are homologous to bulbourethral glands in males. While Bartholin's glands are located in the superficial perineal pouch in females, bulbourethral glands are located in the deep perineal pouch in males.

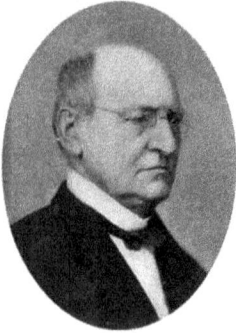

Gurdon Buck
1807-1877

Buck, a leading surgeon in New York City, was known for his method of treating femur fractures using traction produced by a weight and pulley. The deep fascia that encloses the cavernous bodies and the main vessels and nerves of the penis is known as Buck's fascia.

William Cowper
1666-1709

Cowper was an English surgeon. The bulbourethral glands, located adjacent to the membranous urethra in the male, are frequently referred to as Cowper's glands. They empty a secretion into the urethra for the purpose of lubrication.

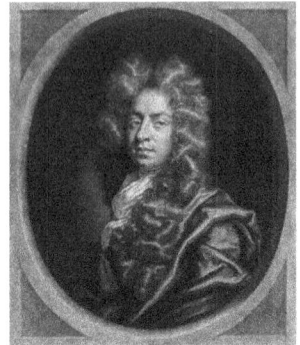

James Douglas
1675-1742

Douglas, a Scotsman, was an anatomist, man-midwife and physician to the queen. In the female, the rectouterine peritoneal pouch is located between the posterior aspect of the uterus and rectum and is commonly referred to as the pouch of Douglas.

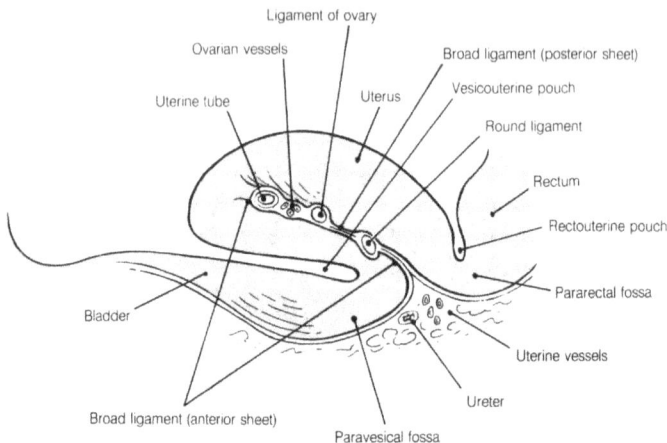

In this midsagittal section of the female pelvis, the space between the rectum and uterus can be seen. It is known as the rectouterine pouch or pouch of Douglas.

Gabriele Falloppio
1523-1563

Falloppio was an Italian anatomist, surgeon and botanist. The uterine tubes are commonly referred to as the Fallopian tubes.

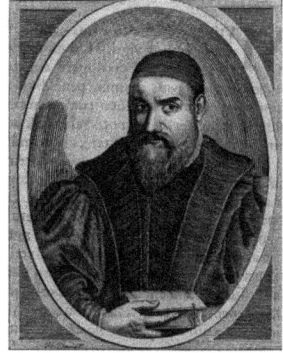

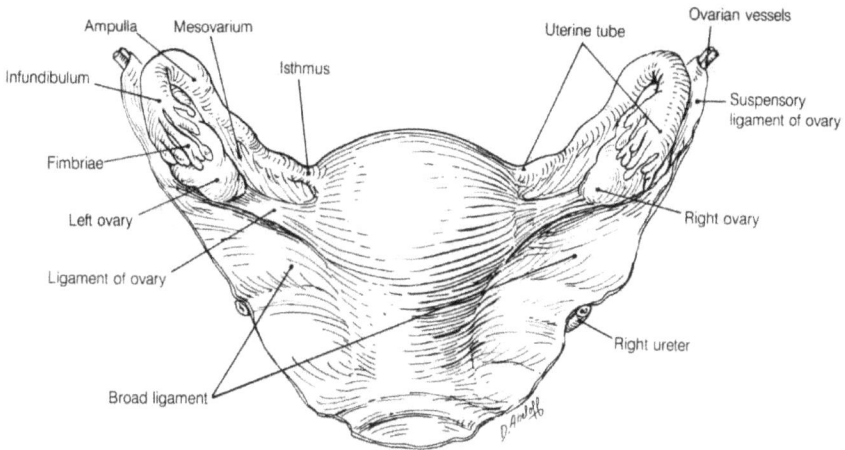

The uterine tubes are more often referred to as Fallopian tubes.

Bern B. Gallaudet
1860-1934

Gallaudet was a prominent professor of anatomy at Columbia University. The deep perineal fascia of the perineum, often known as Gallaudet's fascia, covers the muscles of the superficial perineal pouch, including the bulbospongiosus, ischiocavernosus and superficial transverse perineal muscle.

Hermann Treschow Gartner
1785-1827

Gartner, born in the West Indies, was a surgeon who studied in Denmark and spent his career in Norway, England and Scotland. In the development of the female, the mesonephric tubules and duct develop as part of the urinary system, including the kidney. They then regress, except for parts which persist as the appendix vesiculosa, epoophoron, paroophoron and Gartner's duct.

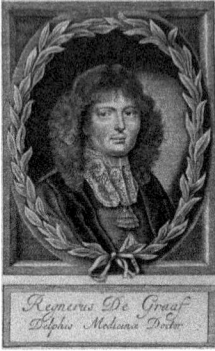

Regnier de Graaf
1641-1673

Graaf was a Dutch anatomist and physician who studied under Franciscus Sylvius. In the ovary, a Graafian or tertiary follicle is the one follicle of a group of secondary follicles that will ovulate.

William Hunter
1718-1783

William Hunter, older brother of John Hunter, was a Scottish physician who operated the School of Anatomy in Covent Garden, London. The University of Glasgow now has his museum and collection of pictures, coins and books. Hunter's eloquent description of the developing fetus in 1774 allowed numerous investigators to refer to the uterine decidua as Hunter's membrane.

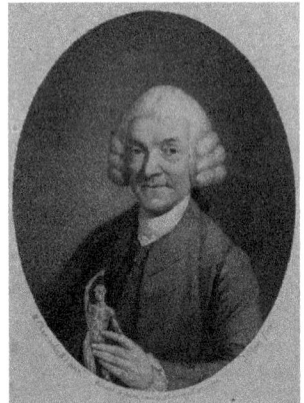

Franz von Leydig
1821-1908

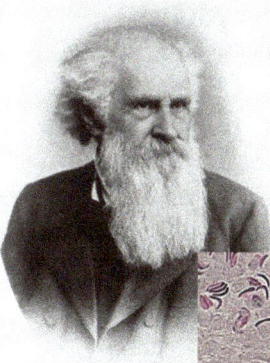

Leydig was a German comparative histologist. The interstitial cells of Leydig in the testis are located in areas between seminiferous tubules and secrete testosterone.

The arrow demonstrates a Leydig cell in the testis. They are known as interstitial cells because they are literally found between or among seminiferous tubules, three of which can been seen at the periphery of this image.

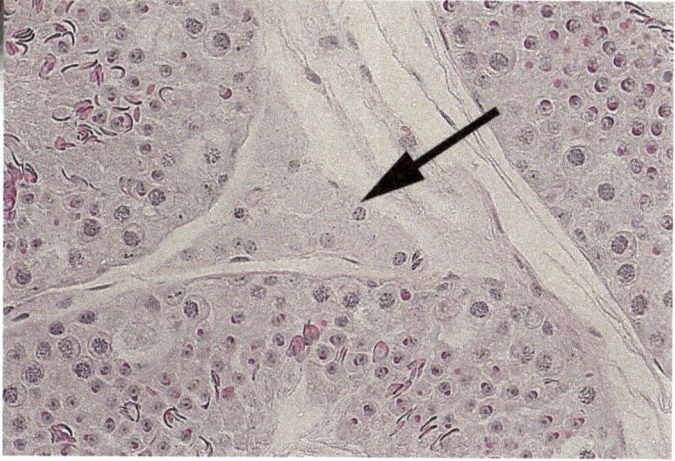

Alwin Mackenrodt
1859-1925

Mackenrodt was a German gynecologist and pathologist. The lateral transverse cervical ligaments of the uterus, sometimes known as the cardinal ligaments, may also be called Mackenrodt's ligaments. They are fibromuscular thickenings of the

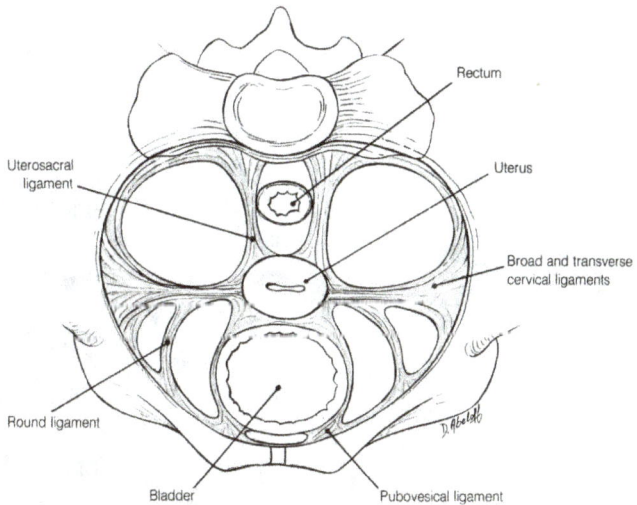

In the female pelvis, the lateral transverse cervical ligaments are known as cardinal ligaments or Mackenrodt's ligaments.

pelvic fascia surrounding the uterine vessels in the base of the broad ligament of the uterus. Attached to the side of the cervix of the uterus and the lateral fornix of the vagina, these ligaments probably play a part in stabilising the uterus and vagina.

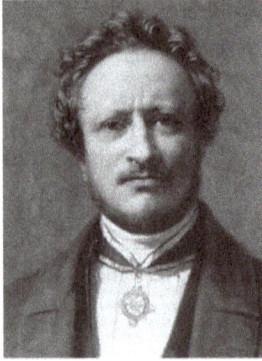

Johannes Peter Muller
1801-1858

Muller was a German anatomist and physiologist. The paramesonephric duct, or Mullerian duct, develops in the embryo from the urogenital ridge and gives rise to the uterine tubes as well as contributing to the development of the broad ligament and vagina.

John A. Sampson
1873-1946

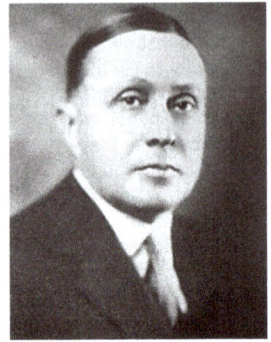

Sampson was a Professor of Gynecology at Albany Medical College in New York. The artery that travels through the round ligament of the uterus represents the anastomosis of the uterine and ovarian arteries and is frequently called Sampson's artery.

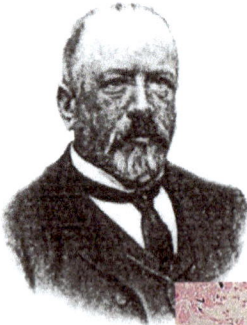

Enrico Sertoli
1842-1910

Sertoli was an Italian professor of physiology. Sertoli cells, located in the epithelium of the seminiferous tubules of the testis, support, nourish and protect the spermatogenic cells.

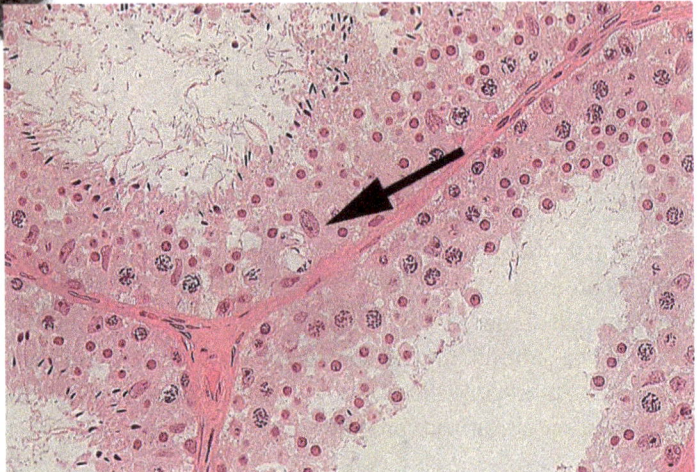

The arrow points out a Sertoli cell within a seminiferous tubule of the testis. The space at the upper left contains numerous small sperm.

AUDITORY SYSTEM

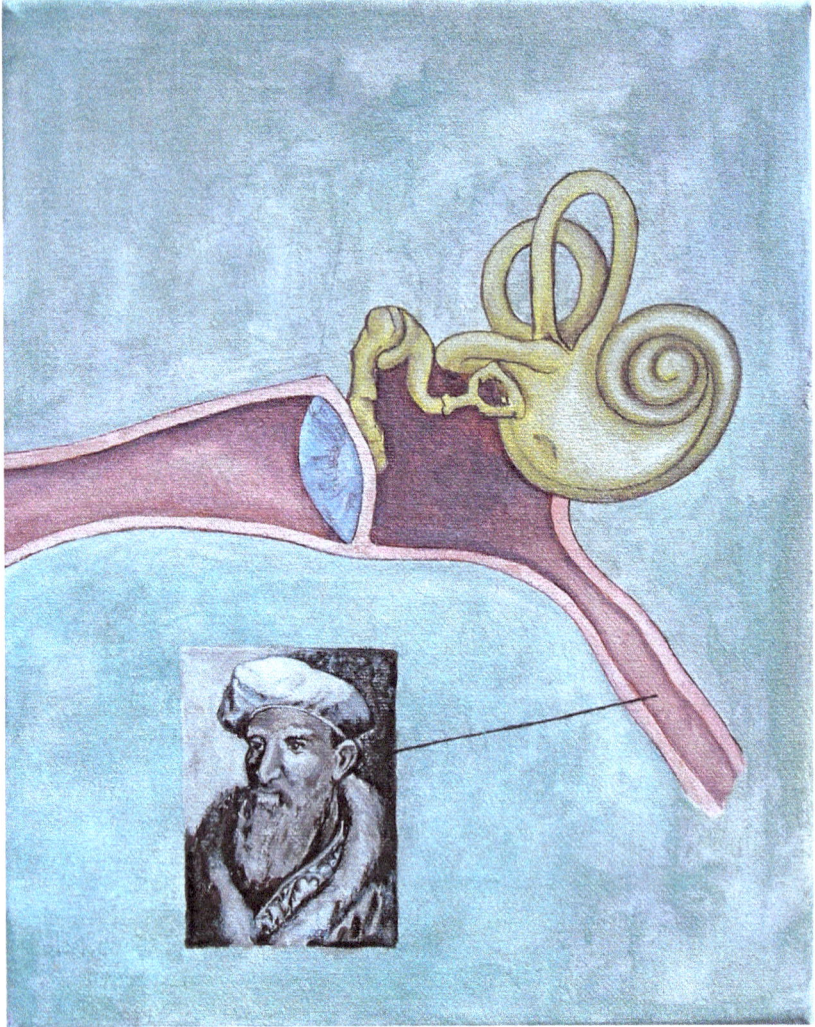

Bartolomeo Eustachi
Taken from *The Alphabet of Anatomical Eponyms* ©Meredith Browne
http://meredithbrowne.weebly.com/alphabet-of-anatomical-eponyms.html

Alfonso Corti
1822-1888

Corti was an Italian histologist who worked in various European cities without ever holding an official academic appointment. In the ear, the cochlear duct contains the spiral organ of Corti in which the receptors of the auditory apparatus are located.

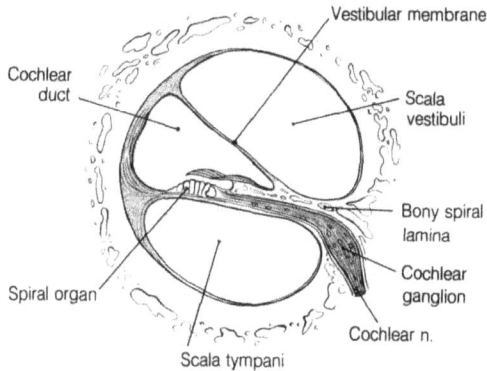

The spiral organ of Corti of the cochlear duct in the internal ear is part of the auditory apparatus.

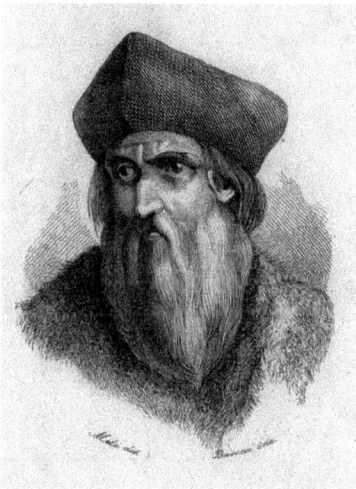

Bartolomeo Eustachi
16th Century

Eustachi, whose birth date is debated, was an Italian physician and anatomist whose anatomical plates were among the first to be produced on copper. The auditory tube, also known as the pharyngotympanic tube, is commonly called the Eustachian tube.

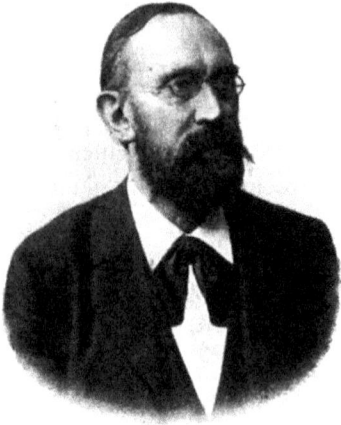

Viktor Hensen
1835-1924

Hensen was a German embryologist and physiologist who studied both the developing embryo and the histology of special sense organs. The tall columnar cells that form the outer border cells of the organ of Corti are commonly called cells of Hensen.

Ludwig Levin Jacobson
1783-1843

Jacobson was an anatomist and physician in Copenhagen, Denmark. The tympanic branch of the glossopharyngeal nerve is often called Jacobson's nerve, and the tympanic plexus is also referred to as Jacobson's tympanic plexus.

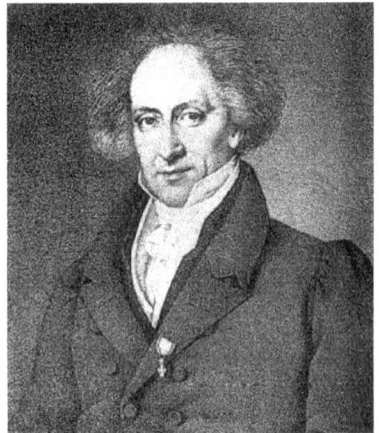

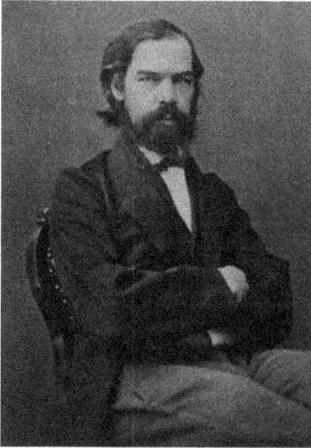

Ernst Reissner
1824-1878

Reissner was an anatomist in Eastern Europe. The vestibular membrane in the cochlear duct is commonly called Reissner's membrane.

The vestibular membrane, also known as Reissner's membrane, is located in the cochlear duct in the internal ear.

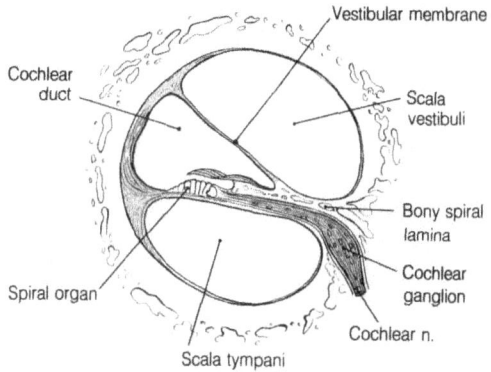

Vestibular membrane

Cochlear duct

Scala vestibuli

Bony spiral lamina

Cochlear ganglion

Cochlear n.

Spiral organ

Scala tympani

VISUAL SYSTEM

Karl Wilhelm Ludwig Bruch
1819-1884

Bruch was a German anatomist. The innermost layer of the choroid that borders directly on the retinal pigment epithelium is known as the lamina vitrea or Bruch's membrane.

Jean Descemet
1732-1810

Descemet was a French anatomist and surgeon. In the cornea, Descemet's membrane is a thick basal lamina that separates the stroma from the endothelium.

Descemet's membrane underlies the corneal endothelium at the tip of the arrow. The space at the top of the image is inside the eye, whereas the space at the bottom of the image is the outside world.

Joseph Ritter von Artha Hasner
1819-1892

Hasner was a Czech anatomist and ophthalmologist. An imperfect valve located at the end of the nasolacrimal duct is called Hasner's valve. It is through this structure that tears from the eye drain into the nasal cavity.

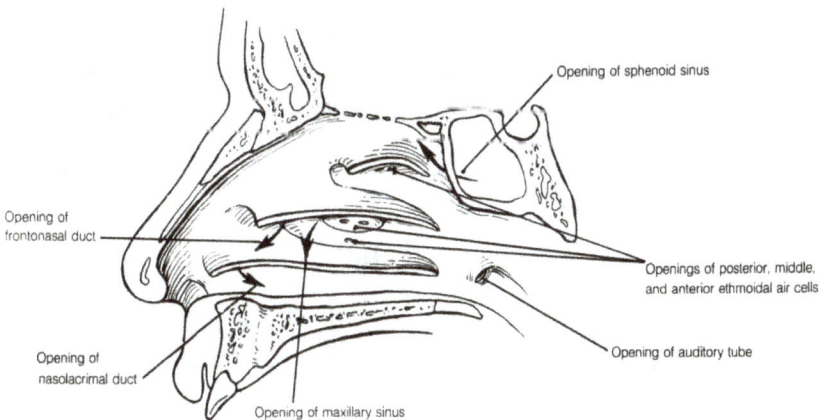

Opening of sphenoid sinus

Opening of frontonasal duct

Openings of posterior, middle, and anterior ethmoidal air cells

Opening of auditory tube

Opening of nasolacrimal duct

Opening of maxillary sinus

The nasolacrimal duct is guarded by Hasner's valve.

Heinrich Meibom
1638-1700

Meibom was a German professor of medicine, history and poetry. Numerous sebaceous glands embedded in the tarsal plate of the upper eyelids are called tarsal or Meibomian glands.

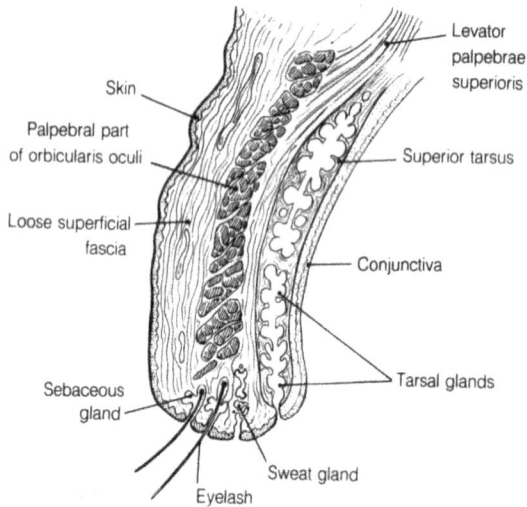

In the upper eyelid are numerous glands known as tarsal glands, or Meibomian glands.

Jacob Antonius Moll
1832-1914

Moll was a Dutch ophthalmologist. The glands of Moll, or ciliary glands, are large modified sweat glands that are located on the edge of the eyelid next to the base of the eyelashes and contribute factors to tears that prevent evaporation (see above).

Heinrich Muller
1820-1864

Muller was a German professor of anatomy. The smooth involuntary muscle of the upper eyelid is known as Muller's muscle.

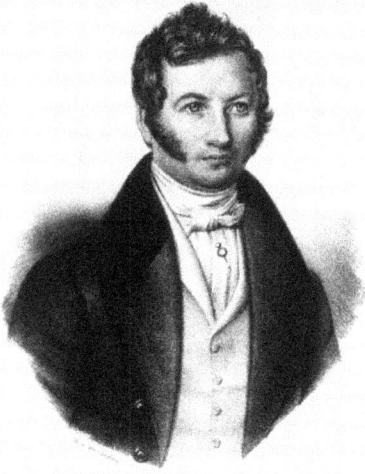

Freidrich Schlemm
1795-1858

Schlemm was a German professor of anatomy. The canal of Schlemm is a circular vascular channel at the junction of the cornea and sclera within the eye. It is through this opening that aqueous humor drains into the venous system. Impaired drainage through this opening leads to increased intraocular pressure and glaucoma.

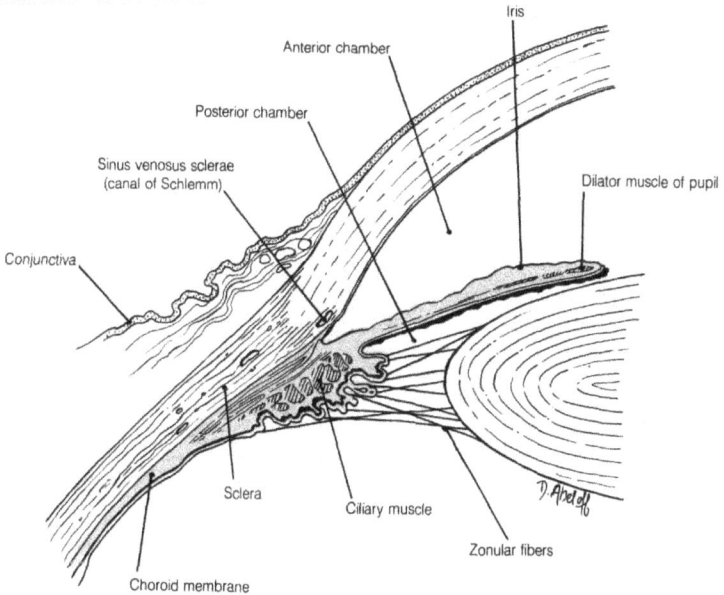

The canal of Schlemm allows drainage of aqueous humor into the venous system.

Jacques Rene Tenon
1724-1816

Tenon was a French army surgeon and professor of pathology who specialised in ophthalmology. The tendons of the eye muscles are attached to the outer surface of the sclera which, in turn, is connected with a dense layer of connective tissue called the capsule of Tenon. The episcleral tissue is continuous with an exceedingly loose system of thin collagenous membranes separated by clefts known as the space of Tenon.

Eduard Zeis
1807-1868

Zeis was an Austrian dermatologist. The ciliary sebaceous glands of the eye are called Zeis's glands.

INDEX OF NAMES

www.ingramcontent.com/pod-product-compliance
Lightning Source LLC
Chambersburg PA
CBHW061258220326
41599CB00028B/5693